D0019568

THE COMPLETE BOOK OF HOMEOPATHY

DR. MICHAEL WEINER
AND
KATHLEEN GOSS

Avery Publishing Group

Garden City Park, New York

THE COMPLETE BOOK OF HOMEOPATHY

Michael Weiner, Ph.D., M.S., M.A.
and
Kathleen Goss

AVERY PUBLISHING GROUP INC.
Garden City Park, New York

This book is not intended to replace your own physician with whom you should consult before taking any medication or considering treatment.

Cover design by Rudy Shur and Martin Hochberg

Library of Congress Cataloging-in-Publication Data

Weiner, Michael A.
    The complete book of homeopathy/
Michael Weiner and Kathleen Goss.
       p. cm.
     Includes index.
     ISBN 0-89529-412-5 : $9.95
     1. Homeopathy. I. Goss, Kathleen. II. Title.
RX71.W45 1989
615.5'32--dc19   88-38463
                                           CIP

Copyright © 1989 by Michael Weiner

All rights reserved. No part of this publication may be reproduced, stored in a retrieval system or transmitted, in any form, by any means, electronic, mechanical, photocopying, recording or otherwise, without the prior permission of the publisher.

Printed in the United States of America

9

CONTENTS

INTRODUCTION

Homeopathy, developed some 170 years ago as a direct reaction against the harmful medical practices of the time, is the original "alternative medicine." With the growth of modern technological medicine, this revolutionary doctrine suffered a setback, but now it appears that America's love affair with technology may be drawing to a close, and that homeopathy's time has finally come.

In the health sciences, there is a growing movement toward a holistic view of the human organism, in which mind is recognized as playing an equal role with material influences in the cause and cure of disease. Whereas the ever-increasing specialization of technological medicine dictates a fragmented approach to treatment, homeopathy has always viewed any illness as a disease of the whole person.

There is also a profound philosophical change taking place in this country—an emerging recognition of the role our individual consciousness plays in mediating our inner experience and our interaction with the environment, and a recognition of consciousness as a means of gaining access to supposedly involuntary biological processes. At the center of the homeopathic doctrine is the concept of the *vital force*, an eloquent statement of the unifying role of individual consciousness. Homeopathic prescribing addresses itself directly to the vital force, viewing it as the key to the organism's self-healing powers.

Patients who have come to distrust the tools of technological medicine—harmful and habit-forming drugs, radiation, chemotherapy, excessive surgery—are now becoming willing to risk discontinuing such treatment and to explore the possibilities of more natural approaches to healing. As people become selective in their patterns of consumption—avoiding processed foods, limiting their use of coffee, tobacco, and alcohol, eliminating the habitual use of over-the-counter drugs—they are preparing their bodies to accept the subtler influences of natural forms of therapeutics, including proper nutrition, exercise, herbs, and homeopathic remedies administered in infinitesimal doses.

In this new climate of open-mindedness, the real test of homeopathy is whether it actually works. Homeopathy was developed as an empirical science, and as such its proof must rest on clinical experience. Although the number of homeopathic practitioners in this country today is small, their case histories are full of examples of the successful application of the homeopathic doctrine. In this book, the reader will have the opportunity to verify that properly selected homeopathic remedies are indeed effective in treating minor illnesses and injuries, and that they offer a more natural alternative to the over-the-counter medications whose dangers are becoming obvious.

It is important for anyone exploring homeopathic remedies to have a clear understanding of the principles on which they operate. Many patients are no longer willing to accept the familiar injunction, "Just take this pill; never mind what it is or what it does." Today's increasingly aware consumers of health care will no longer accept *any* form of medicine on the strength of authority alone; they want to understand the rational basis for their treatment. The present book draws on the classic homeopathic texts as well as the commentaries of modern practitioners to explain the homeopathic doctrine, and it illustrates the principles of homeopathic prescribing with case histories extracted from nearly two centuries of practice.

The proponents of modern technological medicine have objected to homeopathy on the grounds that it is unscientific. As our understanding of the universe continues to evolve, it will become increasingly apparent that homeopathy is more consistent with emerging scientific theory than any other form of medicine, and that this holistic, humane, and natural approach to healing may well be the medicine of the future.

PART I

HOMEOPATHY IN THEORY AND PRACTICE

1

WHY HOMEOPATHY?

THE SEARCH FOR ALTERNATIVES

America's present disillusionment with modern medicine is but one manifestation of a wider concern over the ultimate benefits of modern technology. The products of our research laboratories—food additives, insecticides, drugs with unknown long-term and genetic effects—are threatening our health as rapidly as medical research can unravel the mysteries of disease. The depletion of our energy resources and the unbalancing of our ecology are creating a widespread state of alarm. Current debates over the morality and the dangers of such things as the use of energy or genetic engineering underline a general sense of apprehension that scientists may be interfering with natural processes without being able to predict the consequences of their actions.

Just as environmentalists are questioning the disruption of our ecology, the alternative health movement is seeking ways to treat illness with minimal disruption of the internal environment of the body. This new breed of health practitioner is exploring medical systems that have demonstrated their effectiveness in other cultures for hundreds, even thousands, of years, such as the ancient Chinese system of acupuncture. With cues being taken from both the modern psychological science of learning theory and the time-tested techniques of meditation, it is being found that some therapies—such as biofeedback training—can reeducate an individual to exert conscious control over conditions that may develop into such varied pathology as hypertension, gastric ulcers, and tension headaches. As nutrition comes into its own as a science, health professionals are learning a great deal about the preventive value of a diet that avoids toxic ingredients, and about the curative value of replacing nutritional deficiencies.

Such approaches are relatively new to the Western world. As technological medicine began to make gigantic and impressive strides—with the introduction of wonder drugs such as the antibiotics, with the refinement of diagnostic tools, and with the development of surgical techniques of extraordinary complexity—a number of nonorthodox medical systems that were both relatively harmless and clinically successful were eclipsed. Herbal medicine, practiced since the dawn of man's history and incorporated into a number of popular systems in the nineteenth century, went into a decline and is only now being reexplored for the benefits it can bring to both the sick and the healthy.

Most alternative approaches to health care revolve around a central concept that is as old as the art of healing itself: that each person, each organism, possesses on a deep level the will and wisdom to be healthy, and that the wisdom of the organism can and should be enlisted in effecting a cure.

This belief in the curative wisdom of the body is one of the tenets of homeopathy, a medical system originating in Germany that reached its peak in the United States during the nineteenth century.

Although the word *homeopathy* is becoming familiar once again among those who are interested in nonorthodox medicine, it is still widely misunderstood. Homeopathy is not herbal medicine; nor is it a dietary regimen. It is a philosophy of health and a formal system of drug therapeutics that traces its origins to a single man, Samuel Hahnemann (1755–1843) and was subsequently expanded and elaborated by a number of his followers.

Following the principles laid down by Hahnemann at the beginning of the nineteenth century, homeopaths are able to point to some 170 years of successful practice—without the need for revolutionary revisions of their doctrine and without the need to discover an endless series of new principles upon which to treat disease. The homeopathic practitioner operates on a set of principles that are independent of modern technology and do not require validation by it: the only evidence required for the correctness of the homeopathic doctrine is its actual success in practice.

WHAT'S DIFFERENT ABOUT HOMEOPATHY?

The first thing you will notice if you visit a homeopathic physician is that he goes about treating you in an entirely different way from what you have become accustomed to in orthodox practice. He will spend a great deal of time— perhaps as much as one or two hours—examining you and taking a detailed history of your complaints. He will ask you many things that will surprise you, such as your likes and dislikes in food, in activities, in your dealings with other people. Although he may perform some routine laboratory diagnostic tests, taking blood samples, X rays, and the like, he will make it clear that your treatment will not depend upon a diagnosis based on such test results, but rather upon what he has observed about you during the examination. He will be interested not only in your physical complaints, but also in your mental state and your constitutional responses to such things as changes in weather and other external factors. You will have the feeling that the homeopath is looking at you as an individual; that he is eliciting information that will define you as a distinct person. The purpose of this close questioning is to develop a picture of you that will enable the homeopath to select a remedy that is appropriate for the totality of your symptoms.

We will outline below some of the elements of the homeopathic doctrine that distinguish it from orthodox medicine and, to a greater or lesser degree, from other nonorthodox forms of treatment.

Like Cures Like

Hahnemann called the orthodox medicine of his day *allopathy* from the Greek words *allos* ("different") and *pathein* ("disease, suffering"). To this form of medicine he opposed his system, which he called *homeopathy*, from the Greek *homoion* ("similar") and *pathein* ("disease, suffering"). The key difference between the two systems is summed up in these terms. Today, quite as in Hahnemann's time, orthodox— or allopathic—medicine generally proceeds on the principle that a disease, or a symptom of a disease, is cured by using a medicine that opposes the symptoms—sometimes by direct suppression and sometimes by an indirect route that leads to their removal. A good example is the treatment of pain. In allopathic practice, such drugs as aspirin and opiates are widely used to relieve the patient of pain. Opium works by dulling the central nervous system; the exact mechanism of the action of aspirin is not entirely known, but its end result is to relieve pain. Yet common sense tells us that pain has a value; it is a warning that there is something wrong. If our senses are dulled to the point that we cannot perceive pain, we may suffer serious consequences. Homeopaths use the example of the warning lights on the dashboard of a car: when the oil light comes on, we don't simply disconnect the wire. The light is a signal that there is something wrong in the inner workings of the car, and it is that internal condition that must be corrected. Allopathy proceeds on the principle of administering substances that will remove or alleviate the patient's symptoms without bearing directly on the underlying condition that produced those symptoms.

Partly owing to the influence of the homeopathic example, many branches of modern orthodox medicine now operate on the principle of an inherent similarity between the medicine given and the condition being treated, for example, immunology and replacement therapy in deficiency diseases. However, the vast array of antibiotics, tranquilizers, sleeping medications, laxatives, and antihistamines remain allopathic in their application. Even the descriptive terms for such drugs, full of the prefix "anti-", indicate the principle on which they are prescribed.

The Latin phrase *Similia similibus curantur* ("Like shall be cured by like") forms the cornerstone of the homeopathic doctrine. According to Hahnemann, the proper remedy for an illness is that substance which, in a healthy person, would produce the same set of symptoms exhibited in the sick patient. This Law of Similars was not original with Hahnemann; the idea had been advanced by philosophers and physicians from time to time for thousands of years, and Hahnemann acknowledges his debt to Hippocrates, in whose writings the principle of "like cures like" appears. Hahnemann, however, was the first to build a consistent system of therapeutics based on this principle. In many of the so-called folk medicines of the world, as well as in the writings of the alchemists, there is the Doctrine of Signatures, which holds that each plant intended for use as a medicine contains within itself a sign, or signature, indicating what its use is. Thus the yellow sap of the plant *Chelidonium majus*, or celandine, signifies that it is intended for liver and biliary complaints, since the sap resembles the color of bile. Some of these correspondences prove true in practice; *Chelidonium* is still used by homeopaths and herbalists to treat liver troubles.

Provings of Remedies

Such esoteric indications of the proper uses of plants do not, however, provide sufficient, or reliable, information as to their therapeutic potential. Hahnemann reasoned that in order to know what healing properties are contained in a given substance, we must know what the substance will do in a healthy person, and since Hahnemann's time, a large portion of the work of homeopaths has been the systematic administration of all sorts of substances—derived from the animal, vegetable, and mineral kingdoms—to healthy persons, in order to observe their effects. Such testing of drugs on healthy subjects is known in homeopathy as *proving*.

Although it might strike us as eminently reasonable to determine the effects of drugs by observing their action in healthy people, if we look about us, we can see how drugs are screened for human consumption in orthodox medicine today. Before a new drug is allowed to be used in human experimentation, it is generally tested for a specific action—for example, the killing of certain strains of bacteria—in laboratory animals or simply in isolated cultures. Then, when it is given to humans, it is given to the sick, rather than the healthy. The principal effect sought is the drug's ability to counteract a specific symptom in the sick patient—for example, the reduction of the number of a certain kind of bacteria in the bloodstream. Often, it is not until some years later that physicians become aware of other effects of the drug. Today, just as in Hahnemann's time, it is virtually unheard of to determine the effects of drugs by administering them to healthy people, except for the questionably ethical purpose of determining their toxic levels.

The Single Remedy

The aim of homeopathy is to treat the patient's complex symptom picture with a remedy whose known effects most closely resemble the symptoms of the disease. Homeopathy, therefore, stresses that no more than one remedy is to be given at a time, since the effects of remedies given in combination are unknown. The principle of the single remedy is again in sharp contrast with prevailing orthodox medical practice, in which a patient may leave a doctor's office with prescriptions for half a dozen different drugs, all to be taken at the same time for different complaints, or perhaps even used to counteract the side effects of other drugs. The growth of specialized medical practice often encourages multiple prescriptions, since one specialist will prescribe for one condition and another will prescribe for a different problem.

By insisting on the single remedy, homeopathy reaffirms its insistence on treating the patient as a whole. All the sick person's complaints are examined together, and a single remedy is determined that most nearly matches the whole complex of symptoms. Symptoms are never treated in isolation.

The Minimum Dose and Potentization

Probably the most difficult element of homeopathy for people to accept is its use of extremely small doses of the similar remedy. In Hahnemann's time, it was common practice to treat illness by drastic measures, such as bloodletting, the use of large doses of toxic substances, and the administration of large quantities of purgatives. When Hahnemann first began prescribing on the basis of the Law of Similars, he used the large doses common in his time. Because the remedies he used were known to produce symptoms similar to those from which the patient was suffering, Hahnemann observed that he was causing temporary but sometimes violent aggravations of the patient's symptoms. He began experimenting with reduced doses, and he found that, although the undesirable violent aggravations of the symptoms were reduced, the remedies were still curative. Eventually Hahnemann developed a systematic method of diluting remedies to a point where not even a single molecule of the original medicinal substance might be present in the medication administered to the patient! This process of repeated subdivision and dilution with succussion, or shaking, which is peculiar to homeopathy, is known as *potentization*, since Hahnemann believed that this procedure released hitherto unsuspected curative powers in the medicines thus treated. *The higher the potency of a homeopathic preparation, the smaller the amount of the medicinal substance present in solution.*

For the purpose of a general definition of homeopathy, it is sufficient to say that high-potency preparations are on an order of dilution unheard of in orthodox medical practice and are believed by homeopaths to work on a deeper level than the physiologic sphere of ordinary drugs.

Chronic Diseases

Another theoretical element of homeopathy is Hahnemann's controversial theory of chronic diseases. Hahnemann felt that many acute conditions, as well as recurrent chronic conditions, were actually outcroppings of underlying chronic or constitutional problems, and that these chronic problems had to be cleared up by choosing the most similar remedy from among a group of remedies bearing a strong symptomatic relationship to the underlying illnesses. A patient under homeopathic treatment for a chronic illness may be given only one dose of an extremely high potency, which is allowed a long time to act; it is common for a patient with a troublesome chronic condition not to visit his physician or be given another dose of a remedy for a month, six months, or an entire lifetime. This is in strong contrast with allopathic practice, where many chronic conditions are treated daily with several substantial doses of a medicine, or a combination of medicines, which may never be able to be discontinued.

Theoretically, homeopathy presents an alternative to the high costs and the considerable drug-related risks of modern medicine. It is true that homeopathy cannot treat all conditions: the surgeon still has his rightful place in the homeopathic view, and diseases that have advanced so far as to result in extensive tissue change and organ damage may not respond to homeopathic remedies. But in cases that are susceptible to medical management alone, homeopathy offers an approach to health care that, owing to the minuscule doses given and the well-established effects of the drugs that are used, produces the least possible disturbance within the organism. Homeopaths claim, as well, that patients under homeopathic treatment enjoy an increased resistance to disease, a heightened sense of well-being in their lives, and generally quicker recovery from acute illnesses.

The stage is set today for a rebirth of homeopathy, for many of the problems in modern medicine are strongly reminiscent of the very problems that led Hahnemann to formulate his revolutionary theory.

WHAT'S WRONG WITH MODERN MEDICINE?

With all our modern miracle drugs, our sophisticated surgical procedures, our highly refined diagnostic tools, and our efficient and elaborately instrumented hospitals, the sad truth is that today's medicine may sometimes be no more effective for us than the outdated practices of earlier times. What's more, the very medical techniques in which our civilization takes so much pride are themselves producing new forms of illness, some of which are not recognized until large numbers of people have long been exposed to their hazards.

The potentially dangerous tools of modern medicine are also increasing in cost at an alarming rate. According to a recent television network report, the cost of health care in the United States has risen 1,000 percent since 1950, eight times the rate of increase in the cost of living over the same period. Economic factors alone would seem to justify a search for an alternative approach to health maintenance.

Just as in Hahnemann's time, the problems with today's medicine separate into a few well-defined areas. Setting aside the important question of cost, two major difficulties with modern allopathic medicine can be defined as (1) a rise in iatrogenic, or treatment-induced, disease, and (2) a change in the physician-patient relationship that both grows out of and reinforces a potentially dangerous philosophical orientation to health and illness.

Probably the most visible form of iatrogenic disease in today's society is the result of the often frightening so-called side effects of modern drugs. Let us examine the phrase "side effects." Many of the new drugs were developed for specific purposes, for example, antimicrobials, antihypertensives, sleep-inducing agents, and tranquilizers. Yet the action of these drugs must be sufficiently broad and powerful to produce the desired effect in large numbers of patients who share only one symptom, or group of symptoms, while differing from one another in many other ways. When a powerful drug is given to a broad sample of people, that drug is bound to produce effects over and above the specific one for which it was prescribed. Homeopathic teaching recognizes that drugs have complex, multifaceted effects, as demonstrated in provings on healthy subjects. The proving of any modern drug would similarly elicit a great many symptoms, only one or a few of which would be the effect for which the drug was specifically introduced into the pharmacopoeia.[1] It is a mistake to call these symptoms "side effects," for the side effects are often just as predictable as the antimicrobial, ovulation-suppressing, or antihypertensive effect of the drug. The intended action of a drug, plus its so-called side effects, constitute the symptom complex produced by that drug. When we take an antihistamine for a head cold, we are warned that it may produce drowsiness. The drowsiness is a

1. The *Physicians' Desk Reference,* an annual compendium of manufacturers' descriptions of allopathic drugs, listing their components, dosage, indications for use, and adverse reactions, might actually be considered a summary of the results of provings of these drugs on unwitting subjects.

symptom produced by the drug, just as is the drying out of the mucous membranes, and we must make a choice as to whether we want to be drowsy and have a slight temporary improvement in our nasal congestion, or whether we want to suffer with our stuffy nose and be alert.

Unfortunately, the choices we must make are not always so minor. Even our physicians are not always in a position to make such choices because the facts are not all in. During the 1950s, the hormone diethylstilbestrol was given to large numbers of pregnant women for bleeding during pregnancy or with histories of miscarriages. In 1971, an article in the *New England Journal of Medicine* reported an increased incidence of vaginal cancer in the daughters born to women who had been given the drug.[2]

When such dangerous side effects are suspected, a drug is often taken off the market, as was the case with the tragic discovery that the sedative-hypnotic drug thalidomide induced severe congenital deformities in the children of women who took it during early pregnancy. But in many cases a drug remains in use despite its known dangers. The new broad-spectrum antibiotics are used freely to treat a variety of infectious illnesses, even though they are known to foster the growth of resistant organisms and may have more far-reaching effects:

Predictably, the more powerful antibiotics are much more toxic to human cells and can be as dangerous to life as a generalized infection. Penicillin, the first true antibiotic to be discovered, inter-feres with the cell-wall formation of certain bacteria, and bacterial cell walls (the *outer surfaces* of the cell) are different in important ways from human cell walls. But many newer, more powerful antibiotics are toxic to the basic cellular processes—processes we have in common with bacteria.[3]

There are also subtler forms of iatrogenic illness that arise from unnecessary treatment or unnecessary diagnostic procedures. With the growing number of medical malpractice

2. Herbst, Ulfelder, and Poskanzer, "Adenocarcinoma of the Vagina: Association of Maternal Stilbestrol Therapy with Tumor Appearance in Young Women," *New England Journal of Medicine* 284 (1971):878–81.

3. Andrew Weil, *The Natural Mind* (Boston: Houghton Mifflin Co., 1972), pp. 138–39.

suits, physicians are trying to protect themselves by performing extensive diagnostic procedures that are often unnecessary, as well as risky.

Surgeons today are capable of amazing feats, but many routine surgical procedures, and some not so routine, are of questionable value. Ivan Illich estimates that 90 percent of all tonsillectomies performed in this country are technically unnecessary; that one patient in a thousand dies as a direct consequence of the operation; and that sixteen in a thousand suffer serious complications.[4] All tonsillectomy patients lose the immunity mechanisms the tonsils provide. It is true that orthodox medicine is taking a critical look at the need for tonsillectomy, and the number of such procedures performed annually has decreased over the past few years, yet a significant percentage of American children—20 to 30 percent— still undergo the operation.

So dependent have we become upon the judgment of our physicians that we allow ourselves to be subjected to painful, disease-producing, and disabling procedures and drug treatment, although statistics show that these forms of intervention are often without effect. For example, despite the $500 million a year that the U.S. government now spends on cancer research, as well as the vast sums spent by cancer patients, the forms of therapy used in many types of cancer do not seem to have a significant effect on the patient's survival rate.[5]

We have seen occasional examples of how doctors have caused unintentional harm to the health of a patient by intervening in an often minor illness only to inflict a more serious long-term illness or disability. Yet perhaps the most destructive effect of modern orthodox medicine lies in the changes that have taken place in the relationship between physician and patient. With the advent of medical specialization, the patient is treated as a fragmented being; she goes to the gynecologist for problems with her pelvic organs, to the orthopedist for backache and muscle and joint pains, to the psychiatrist for emotional disturbances. The general

4. Ivan Illich, *Medical Nemesis* (New York: Bantam Books, 1977), p. 106.
5. Ibid., pp. 15–16.

practitioner is all but a thing of the past, and each specialist treats only that organ system that comes within his area of expertise. No wonder we feel that our doctors are not really looking at us as whole beings. Common sense tells us that many symptoms appearing in different organ systems may be related—that they at least constitute a whole picture of our state of health. Yet our trips to the doctor's office must often result in a sense of frustration when we feel that the specific organ-directed treatment we receive is not based on the doctor's assessment of our entire symptom picture.

As medical technology proliferates, we lose the personal contact with the family doctor that was undoubtedly a significant element of the healing process. Fluids and tissue samples are removed from our bodies and analyzed by machinery; the complaint that we don't feel right appears to go unheard unless laboratory tests reveal a deviation from an arbitrarily defined normal range that fits into a diagnostic category.

The growth of assembly-line medicine has done more than destroy the therapeutic milieu of the family doctor's office; through a series of subtle readjustments in the doctor-patient relationship, it has caused the patient to surrender responsibility for his health. Many people rush to the hospital emergency room with every little ailment, not trusting their own judgment as to whether an illness is serious or not. Others rush to the over-the-counter pharmaceutical industry and dose themselves with whatever drug promises the swiftest relief from headache, insomnia, indigestion, constipation, or cold symptoms. They do not trust the wisdom of their own bodies to restore their health.

Despite the fact that medicine has developed spectacular new drugs and techniques, the evidence suggests that we are not any healthier. Many of the old epidemic diseases, such as scarlet fever, whooping cough, diphtheria, cholera, typhoid, polio, and measles, have been brought under control. Although the development of powerful antibiotics and effective vaccines has been a major factor, it is highly probable that an important contributor to the reduction of these diseases is the improved sanitation of modern industrialized nations. But we are now seeing other diseases in epidemic proportions: heart disease, emphysema, cancer, arthritis, hypertension, diabetes, mental illness. It is not enough to explain such new epidemics as "diseases of aging" that have increased in incidence because more people are living longer; cancer is on the increase among children as well as adults, and it is now the second leading cause of death among children.

The homeopathic analysis of these trends projects a frightening view. Homeopathy holds that the epidemic nature of these chronic diseases is a direct result of the suppression of symptoms through modern, allopathic techniques. By suppressing or palliating the symptoms of disease—tumors, blocked blood vessels, measurable high blood pressure—physicians are allowing the underlying causes to progress unseen, thereby making ever more destructive inroads on the human body.

The above discussion of the dangers of modern allopathic medicine may sound unnecessarily harsh. We have all known doctors who have been genuinely concerned about our health, and we have all been relieved of the symptoms of illness by taking allopathic medications. Although it is undeniably true that organized medicine, together with the pharmaceutical and hospital industries, has a virtual stranglehold on the health of our nation today, we do not mean to indict the individual practitioner who is doing the best he can. Many doctors, themselves concerned about the dangerous effects of the drugs they have at their disposal, exercise admirable caution in prescribing; many surgeons take up the scalpel only when it is absolutely necessary. Many physicians are also aware of the limitations of their education and are actively seeking information in areas that the medical school curriculum covers incompletely or not at all, such as nutrition and nondrug therapies including psychosomatic healing, massage, and acupuncture. But many well-intentioned doctors are working under a severe handicap: they have had the underlying assumptions of allopathy drilled into them through their years of medical internship, residency, and clinical practice, and they are inundated by the highly sophisticated advertising put out by the pharmaceutical industry.

Allopathic medicine has a well-defended blind spot when it comes to evaluating the claims of homeopathy. Since the beginnings of homeopathic practice, orthodox physicians have flatly denied that it works, although the lore of homeopathy is full of stories of the conversions of allopaths who set out to disprove Hahnemann's doctrine and ended up embracing it when they observed its results. Hopefully, as the alternative health movement grows, open-minded allopaths will have the opportunity to observe the benefits of nonorthodox therapies (as has already been the case, for example, with acupuncture) and will subject them to clinical trial.

THE HOLISTIC PHILOSOPHY UNDERLYING HOMEOPATHY

Today, as in Hahnemann's time, the dangers of orthodox medical treatment can be traced in part to its focusing on isolated symptoms to the exclusion of all the other facets of the patient's state of well-being. Similarly, orthodox medicine does not individualize the patient, but treats him as a "case" of a "disease," without regard for those aspects of the patient that differentiate him from all other cases of the same "disease."

The contemporary holistic health movement is a modern expression of a strong tradition that has pervaded medicine since the writings of Hippocrates in the fourth century B.C. Harris Coulter, in his three-volume historical work, *Divided Legacy*, analyzes the development of Western medicine in terms of a schism between the tradition of rationalism, which has generally been the dominant form, and empiricism, under which the holistic approach can be subsumed. Although the empiricists have generally represented the minority view in medicine, their original thought and strict reliance on the evidence of experience have made them a potent influence on the mainstream.

Throughout medical history, the rationalists have based their practice on abstract, deductive theory; and as theories changed, so did treatment. Focusing on theoretical considerations of the causes of disease, the rationalists have often lost sight of the patient. The empiricists, on the other hand, base their practice on observation and experience; the patient as an individual is the focus of their therapeutic concerns, and the empirical practitioner treats the patient, according to what is actually observed, rather than the disease, whose cause can only be inferred through abstract reasoning.

Holism, from the Greek word *holos* ("a whole"), is a philosophic theory based on the idea that a whole cannot be analyzed without residue into the sum of its parts. The holistic health movement today comprises many different approaches to healing, including acupuncture, naturopathy, nutrition, herbalism, various systems of exercise, as well as homeopathy. Although the channels through which therapy is applied may differ, the holistic disciplines share a set of assumptions about the nature of health and disease.

Health and Disease

Health, according to the holistic view, is something that can be defined in a positive way. Orthodox medicine, probably because it has developed such a highly impersonal, technologized way of looking at the human organism, has fallen into the habit of defining health simply as the absence of disease. Of course, extended far enough, this definition would encompass everything that we intuitively consider to be health; but, with the high degree of specialization in modern medicine, it is difficult for the average physician to recognize disease itself outside the narrowly defined diagnostic categories that he has learned to identify and treat.

There is a trend in orthodox medicine, though somewhat nominal at present, toward educating medical students to adopt a holistic definition of health. Even such a prominent medical group as the World Health Organization has defined health as a state of complete physical, mental, and social well-being, rather than merely the absence of illness or infirmity, and it is this integrated functioning of the mental, physical, and emotional aspects of the individual that we intuitively recognize as health.

Physicians in ancient China were paid when their patients were healthy and not paid when they were sick. By thus defining the social and economic role of the physician, the Chinese guaranteed that their medical system was health oriented, rather than disease oriented. In contemporary allopathic practice, we all too often see medicine intervening only in crisis situations, doing nothing to preserve health on an ongoing preventive basis.

The harmonious functioning of body, mind, and spirit that we have defined as health is a state of freedom: freedom to carry out the activities of our daily lives; freedom to work and play, to reflect, to socialize with our fellow human beings; even the freedom to accept the yoke of religious constraints. Anything within us that prevents us from exercising our inherent freedom as thinking and willing organisms is, according to this holistic doctrine, illness.

A corollary to these definitions is that disease, an imbalance of the integrated functioning of the organism, is expressed not only on the physical plane, but also on the mental and emotional planes. Orthodox medicine has come to recognize the connection between mental and physical states, acknowledging that a wide variety of complaints—such as gastrointestinal problems, cardiac symptoms, even disabling musculoskeletal disorders—may have psychic components. Similarly, it is now being recognized that many physical illnesses have concomitant mental symptoms that must also be treated. Unfortunately, despite this awareness of the linking of the mental and physical components of disease, orthodox medicine continues to treat the patient on allopathic principles, suppressing the physical symptom, or its inferred psychic cause, or both.

As we shall see, illness cannot afflict the individual solely through physical causes (except in the case of gross trauma); there must be some inner factor, some state of susceptibility, that makes us subject to disease-causing influences. Susceptibility, according to the holistic view, cannot be defined in purely physical terms; it reflects the deepest levels of our being, where the nonphysical plays an important role. In large part, the holistic health disciplines, including homeopathy, aim to maintain health by reducing susceptibility to disease-producing influences. Orthodox medicine similarly recognizes the need to move into the sphere of preventive medicine, but at present this is largely a utopian goal, and efforts in this direction are limited by orthodoxy's materialistic orientation.

The Healing Power of Nature

A second precept of holistic medicine is that there is an inherent tendency in all living things to respond in a self-curative manner toward illness. This healing force is nature, the *vis medicatrix naturae*, has been acknowledged by writers since earliest times, and it is one of the cornerstones of contemporary holistic health practice. We observe this healing power at work in animals when they are sick: they will sleep more or change their diets—acts conducive to the restoration of health. A sick animal in the wild will seek out and eat the specific plant that will remedy its particular illness.

Unfortunately, modern man seems to have lost some of those miraculous instincts that lead the sick animal to the proper plant. Perhaps it is simply that man can no longer act on his instincts, since his food sources have become so sharply delimited by the necessities of urban civilization and technological agriculture. Furthermore, man has contaminated his environment with toxic materials which undoubtedly interfere with the harmonious self-curative forces of nature; and he has contaminated his own body, over generations, with drugs that may have implanted new forms of disease and maladaptation within the organism.

At the same time that man has developed an increasingly technologized civilization, his brain has evolved beyond the level of the other primates. Our highly evolved brains permit us to benefit not only from our own experience, but also from the experience of our forebears and of others around us. It would not seem out of place to say that our ability to observe, recall, compare, reflect, and infer—from sense data immediately before us, from our own store of memories and sensations, and from the written record of the rest of humankind—may be a compensating expression of the aforementioned healing power. Thus, man has shown the capability of developing systems of therapeutics—based on observation, reflection, and experimentation—that can supplement the instinctual processes that maintain and restore health. According to this view, the aim of medical treatment is to stimulate the reactive healing forces of the organism.

The Unknowability of Underlying Processes

In spite of our ability to reason, we can never hope to know with certainty the nature of ultimates. As modern science progresses, this unknowability actually becomes a factor in complex computations. Witness the uncertainty principle in quantum mechanics: the closer we get to analyzing the constituents of the atom or to observing the movement and change that occur among the galaxies, the more are we forced to recognize that there is something beyond our acquired knowledge that is not knowable by ordinary means. The very instruments we use impose a limitation on what kind of information we can obtain.

It would be presumptuous for a scientist to claim that he could point to the precise physical cause of a disease. Bodily processes are understood in a number of distinct, narrowly defined terms—biochemistry, neurophysiology, fluid dynamics, endocrinology, and so forth—but there is no unifying theory in medicine that interrelates all these ways of looking at the living human organism. Just as with the atom, we cannot look into the human body to study disease without imposing limits on what we will see. Furthermore, most of the ways we have of looking into the body can destroy, or do serious damage to, the life within. X rays have been widely used to look into the body in a presumably harmless way; even shoe stores had fluoroscopes so that customers could see how the bones in their feet adapted to their new footgear. Now we know that exposure to X rays can have an injurious effect on living tissue.

If our technology will not permit us to investigate the ultimate underlying mechanisms of disease and health, we can learn even less from pure conjecture. Empty theorizing, without evidence based on observation and experience, is of little value in curing illness.

When we look closely into some of our ideas about disease, we notice that they leave a great deal unexplained. Over the last century, our culture has taught us to believe in the germ theory of disease. With the force of religious dogma, an almost morbid fear of invisible "bugs" creeping around on our unwashed hands was instilled in us during childhood. Yet if a certain kind of bacteria causes a certain disease, why is it that, when we are exposed to a sick person, some of us will get sick and others won't? We all have bacteria living on and inside our bodies at all times—often the same strains of bacteria that are associated with the diseases with which we sometimes fall ill. What conditions are conducive to such bacteria beginning to reproduce out of control? If it isn't something that the bacteria themselves do, it must be something within us that changes, thus disturbing the usually harmless balance between us and these germs. Increased numbers of certain kinds of bacteria are demonstrably associated with certain kinds of illness; this does not mean that the bacteria are the sole cause of the illness. The holistic disciplines generally view bacterial overgrowth as a product of, rather than a cause of, disease. This means that the real disease must be something internal, and possibly immaterial, that we have no way of perceiving directly with our microscopes and our analysis of body fluids and tissues.[6]

Sources of Knowledge about Disease

Given the unknowability of the ultimate nature of disease, we must rely for our information only upon those things we can actually observe, or those things that are reported to the doctor by the patient. Observable phenomena include the signs and symptoms of illness—all those changes in the body that can be seen by the doctor in a physical examination: skin changes, localized pain, changes in reflexes and functions, etc. They also include what the doctor observes about the patient's state of mind—such as her agitated or comatose condition, her movements—and what the patient reports about her inward state, that is, how she *feels*. Modern laboratory tests can give us the various chemical and biological constituents of our body fluids; tissue change can be observed under the microscope; radioactive dye can be injected into a

6. This denial that microorganisms are the sole cause of disease should not be taken to imply that we shouldn't exercise normal precautions in hygiene. As the professor of psychosomatic medicine cautioned his zealous graduates, "Gentlemen, we must remember, microbes *do* exist!"

vein and its course traced through the body by means of a radiosensitive scanner. We have all these tools of modern pathology at our disposal, and the findings of such procedures might be included in the category of symptomatology; however, the holistic health disciplines tend to place less value on laboratory diagnostic procedures and more on the doctor's observations and the patient's report about how she feels.

Homeopathy views symptoms of illness as an expression of the healing power of nature rather than as undesirable "wounds" inflicted on the organism by the disease process.

Rejection of the "Disease Entity"

One of the sharpest points of contrast between the holistic approach and orthodox medicine lies in the difference in emphasis on making a diagnosis.

Before the orthodox physician can prescribe for his patient, he must assign a diagnostic name to the disease from which the patient suffers. Allopathic treatment groups patients according to the diagnosis they share; even though there may be striking differences among patients in the way they react to a given illness, they will all be treated similarly if they are diagnosed as having the same disease. Diagnostic names are assigned to conditions in which certain kinds of symptoms—such as tissue or organ changes, changes in the chemical composition of the blood, or the presence of certain bacteria—are found to be present, regardless of the many things that may distinguish one patient with such symptoms from another. Because diagnosis precedes treatment in allopathic practice, the patient may need to undergo extensive laboratory and pathological tests to be sure he has a certain disease before treatment can be initiated. The rapid acceptance by allopathic medicine of broad-spectrum antibiotics and other drugs is due in part to the need to treat the patient immediately, without waiting for the results of elaborate batteries of diagnostic tests.

In the holistic approach, it is not necessary to determine the disease from which the patient suffers, since treatment can begin on the basis of symptoms alone and is determined by the picture of the patient as a whole and as an individual rather than by the similarity of his illness to that of other people with whom he may share some symptoms in common. To fulfill the requirements of record keeping, or in order to discuss the patient's ailment with him and his family, the holistic practitioner may say that the patient is suffering from a "kind of flu" or a "kind of ulcerative disease," but such names do not by themselves determine the treatment the patient will receive; they simply make the illness more comprehensible in laymen's terms.

Diagnostic names can be misleading. After all, they merely represent an arbitrary selection of certain manifestations of illness that appear together with a certian degree of frequency. The entire methodology of diagnosis has been expanded and refined considerably through the application of modern statistical techniques, but the resulting diagnostic categories represent nothing more than that—statistical groupings of certain kinds of symptoms that tend to occur in combination.

So strongly has the notion of diagnosis become ingrained into allopathic thinking that orthodox physicians often refer to diagnostic categories as "disease entities," as if the diseases had lives of their own, independent of the people whom they affect. The notion of the disease entity tends to reinforce the allopathic attitude that all symptoms of illness are wounds inflicted by an external disease-producing cause rather than expressions of the vital principle in the organism that is trying to throw off the influence of illness. The allopathic focus on treating the disease rather than the individual patient lies at the heart of much of our present dissatisfaction with orthodox medicine. In the course of combating the disease, the allopath may lose sight of the integrity of the patient; and we see many patients today subjected to painful, demoralizing treatment, such as chemotherapy and radiation therapy in cancer, artificial life support in terminal cases, and endless rounds of surgery. The terminal patient's body often becomes a virtual battleground in which allopathy marshals all its resources against a poorly understood antagonist, and the patient is deprived of the option of making his final peace with the world with his mind and body relatively intact.

Homeopathy as a Holistic Approach

The word *holistic* is being used loosely today to refer to a large number of different therapies that share the assumption that illness is a disturbance of the patient as a whole, encompassing not only the physical but also the mental and emotional planes. The holistic health movement actually comprises a number of different therapies, and it constitutes a pluralistic approach to the maintenance of the balanced functioning of the organism. Many of the holistic disciplines can be valuable adjuncts to regular medical treatment or can supplement one another.

Many of the ways of reaching and stimulating the self-curative forces of the organism require a regimen of discipline on the part of the individual: various systems of exercise, the regulation of body functions through dietary control, or deliberate self-programming through biofeedback or meditative techniques. These can only be successful if the individual adheres to the regimen prescribed. In other systems, the "patient" is relatively passive and is operated upon by the healer, as in systems of massage or acupuncture. Although such systems have enormous benefits in improving the general state of well-being of the individual, they are not suited to people whose state of health is dangerously poor, either because of an acute crisis or because of a deep-seated deteriorating chronic condition.

In order to treat the seriously ill patient, it is necessary to effect a profound change on the deepest levels. Homeopathy represents a way of intervening at the level of the patient's reactive, self-curative powers, with or without the patient's full cooperation, to bring about a change in the total functioning of the organism. Although homeopathic treatment can be supplemented by other holistic therapies, it claims to be able to stand alone in effecting such a profound change.

In this sense it is truly holistic, for, through the administration of medicines carefully selected to match the patient's total symptomatology, it can deal equally well with disorders of the body, the mind, and the emotions.

Keeping in mind the implicit philosophical framework of the holistic approach, let us now examine the details of the homeopathic doctrine that distinguish it from other holistic therapies.

2

PRINCIPLES OF HOMEOPATHY

This chapter will present the most important principles of homeopathic theory as stated in the classic homeopathic texts and as practiced by contemporary homeopathic prescribers. If you are the patient of a homeopathic practitioner, or if you are considering going to one, the information here will be enough to give you a clear idea of why the homeopath does things the way he does.

There are a number of books available that provide information on homeopathic self-prescribing. Although the following discussion of homeopathic principles is considerably more extensive than what is given in many introductory manuals, bear in mind that this is not an instruction manual but rather a survey of the theory and practice of homeopathy as it is available in the United States today. Many people will undoubtedly want to test the homeopathic doctrine by trying homeopathic remedies on themselves. Although chapter 3 does discuss how certain remedies are used in first aid situations and in a few minor illnesses, the reader is warned that most self-prescribing should be done with the guidance of far more extensive reference materials, and preferably under the direction of a homeopathic physician. If the reader wants to make a serious investigation of the effects of homeopathic remedies, any of the books listed in Appendix A would be a good place to begin study along these lines.

Some of the principles of the homeopathic doctrine have been the subject of heated dispute, not only between allopaths and homeopaths, but also within the ranks of homeopathy itself, and in subsequent portions of this book we shall be looking at some of the controversial aspects to see how these issues are resolved by contemporary homeopaths in actual practice.

What Is Curable in Diseases

We have seen that homeopathy views tissue changes as the results of disease rather than as disease itself. Certain pathological changes in the sick person are so far advanced that they cannot be considered curable by medicine; for example, a badly decayed tooth cannot be restored to its normal healthy condition. Knowing what is curable in disease requires a thorough familiarity with illness as it manifests itself both in the individual and in humanity as a whole. Homeopathy does not rely on disease names in the same way as allopathy; nevertheless, the doctor should be familiar with the way certain clearly defined kinds of illnesses manifest themselves among the general population. In each individual case of a specific disease, the doctor will see a somewhat different group of symptoms, and by comparing the totality of the symptoms presented by the individual patient with the overall symptom picture that characterizes a certain type of disease, the homeopathic physician will be guided in his selection of a remedy. It is obvious that this knowledge of diseases must come from thorough medical training and extensive clinical experience with the sick.

A great many apparent illnesses, which in homeopathy may be called *indispositions*, are brought on by external factors only—errors in the habits of living, environmental factors, or business worries—and will disappear if the cause of the indisposition is removed. A discerning physician will recognize the external causes in these cases and will simply try to remove them where possible.

Another class of illnesses must be recognized as requiring the attention of a surgeon. Although homeopaths have been able to cure a great many cases of appendicitis, kidney stones, and the like simply through the use of homeopathic remedies, homeopathy fully recognizes the importance of surgical intervention in a variety of cases, for example, fractures and organic changes not susceptible to medical management. Until the surgical condition is corrected, the patient will not be able to respond to the homeopathic remedy that will restore him to complete health.

One of the most troublesome kinds of disease encountered by the contemporary homeopath is the chronic illness resulting from the use of allopathic drugs. Homeopaths trace some chronic conditions back to vaccination in the distant past, or to the suppression of symptoms through the incautious use of local medications, antibiotics, and other drugs that remove surface symptoms but do nothing to remove the internal cause of a disease. Some cases have been so badly mixed up through improper use of drugs that they may actually be incurable; in all such cases of chronic drug disease, the homeopath must proceed with the utmost caution in order not to further complicate the case.

Acting in a preventative manner, the homeopathic physician will also attempt to eliminate those elements of the patients' life that derange health. Counseling on diet, exercise, proper hygiene, and the cessation of injurious habits all fall into this category. Thus, even before he has made use of his vast armamentarium of drugs, the homeopathic physician is in a position to do the patient a great deal of good. Many systems of healing work primarily on this level of health maintenance, and from the enthusiasm and success with which people adhere to various systems of diet, exercise regimens, and the like, we see that these simple precautions can go a long way toward keeping us healthy.

What Is Curative in Medicines

The physician must also know what curative powers lie in the medicines at his disposal, and the experimental search for information about the curative properties of a multitude of medicines has occupied a great deal of the time and thought of the homeopaths. Unlike allopathic medicine, which derives most of its knowledge of drugs from experiments on animals and tests with sick patients, homeopathy reasons that drugs must be tested, or "proved," on healthy subjects, since it is only in the healthy person that the drug has the chance to express itself in its pure form, unmitigated by interaction with a disease process. The innovative quest for knowledge about drugs through provings on healthy subjects has yielded a fascinating body of literature.

Principles for the Use of Medicine in Illness

The homeopathic doctrine is essentially a set of principles to guide the physician in his selection of the proper medicine to treat each individual patient. Once the physician has ascertained what is to be cured in the patient, and once he knows what effects each of his drugs produces upon the human economy, he still needs a consistent, rational set of rules upon which to base his use of these medicines. Although homeopathy is based on certain assumptions about the nature of health and disease, the central concern of homeopathy is the practical question of how to use drugs to treat disease. Homeopathy is thus a medical specialty that builds on the knowledge the physician has gained through his basic medical education. A homeopath may have specialized knowledge of surgery, nutrition, or other areas, but what makes him a homeopathic physician is his application of the formal system of drug therapeutics first laid down by Hahnemann and followed consistently by homeopaths to the present day.

VITAL FORCE

Underlying the specific precepts of homeopathy there is a vitalistic principle that is clearly spelled out by Hahnemann in the opening pages of his *Organon of Medicine*:

In the healthy condition of man, the spiritual vital force (autocracy), the dynamis that animates the material body (organism), rules with unbounded sway, and retains all the parts of the organism in admirable, harmonious, vital operation, as regards both sensations and functions, so that our indwelling, reason-gifted mind can freely employ this living, healthy instrument for the higher purposes of our existence.

The material organism, without the vital force, is capable of no sensation, no function, no self preservation.

It is dead, and now only subject to the power of the external world; it decays, and is again resolved into its chemical constituents.[1]

When we are healthy, we are capable of all the normal functions of life—reaction to our environment, thought and creative action, social and economic interaction with our fellow humans—solely because we are animated by this inner dynamic principle.

This vitalistic principle at the heart of the homeopathic doctrine distinguishes it from the materialistic orientation of orthodox medicine. As we have seen, the vitalistic concept of the healing power of nature is a characteristic element of the holistic approach to health. It has taken many forms in the world's philosophies, for example, the Ch'i in Chinese thought, prana or kundalini in Indian literature, and the orgone of Reichian theory.

The idea of the vital force has important implications for the treatment of illness. In orthodox medicine, the attempt to reduce diagnosis to the identification of material causes—such as germs, viruses, disturbances in chemical balances—leads to a form of treatment directed against these material things. Likewise, orthodox medicine places great importance on the study of pathological changes in the body—the microscopic study of tissues, analysis of the chemical composition of the blood, etc. Because homeopathy views illness as a dynamic disturbance of the vital force, such material evidence of disease is considered the result of disease rather than its cause, although this does not mean that the homeopath completely disregards such pathologic data.

The Meaning of Symptoms

In the homeopathic view, the symptoms of illness—the changes in the sensations and functions of the organism that are perceptible to the patient or to the physician—are the only information we can hope to obtain about the true nature of a

1. Samuel Hahnemann, *Organon of Medicine*, trans. with Preface by William Boericke, M.D., and Introduction by James Krauss, M.D. (New Delhi: B. Jain Publishers, 1976), section 9–10 and note. There are many editions of the *Organon*; all quotations herein will be from the edition cited here.

disease. They are also the visible expression of the vital force reacting against the disease process. Since orthodox medicine views symptoms as being inflicted on the organism by a disease cause, the symptoms, seen as evidence of a morbid process, must be eradicated or suppressed by such means as are available to the allopathic doctor.

In homeopathy, symptoms are seen as expressions of a curative process—the organism's attempts, however ineffectual in some cases, to heal itself. Taking cues from the reactive expression of the vital force, the homeopathic physician seeks to promote the symptoms, thereby stimulating the reactive vital force and helping to complete the curative process that has already been set in motion.

A simple example of the difference between the homeopathic and the allopathic way of looking at symptoms is the treatment of fever. We Americans consume vast quantities of over-the-counter allopathic medicines, such as aspirin and acetaminophen, that reduce fever. Very high fevers can certainly be dangerous, but at the slightest hint of an above-normal temperature, the common response is to start taking aspirin to bring the fever down. Folk wisdom and the analysis of many holistic medical philosophies throughout the ages teach that fever is nature's way of dealing with certain morbific influences. The great alchemist Paracelsus and his followers in the empiricist tradition spoke of *coction*, or "cooking out" of the disease-causing influences. Mothers through the ages have breathed a sigh of relief when their sick children ran a high fever with sweating, knowing that the crisis was about to pass. When the body temperature is raised a few degrees, the internal environment is radically changed and becomes no longer hospitable to certain bacteria; eliminative processes may then proceed at an increased rate, and the body, through its own wisdom, functions to heal itself.

Another example may be observed in the treatment of what is known as hay fever. Orthodox medicine sees the runny nose and other exits for mucus as disturbing factors. The homeopath interprets these symptoms as the flow of waste products necessary to rid the organism of offending pollen. Thus the allopath prescribes antihistamines or ephedrine compounds to suppress symptoms, forcing the sufferer to retain substantial amounts of proteinaceous pollen that may continue to irritate and disturb the patient long after the flowering season has passed.

The natural discharges of the body—urine, sweat, menses, feces, skin eruptions—are an important means by which the organism rids itself of waste substances and toxic materials. These discharges help maintain the normal balance of functions—ingestion and excretion; anabolism (assimilation and building up) and catabolism (breaking down). The allopathic physician will often attempt to suppress one or another of these discharges. He will give a medication to control diarrhea, or, even more commonly, to suppress skin eruptions. Since the homeopath views such discharges as the organism's way of ridding itself of toxic substances, in homeopathy the suppression of such discharges is considered particularly dangerous, possibly leading to more serious chronic conditions.

Acute and Chronic Diseases

According to the vitalistic concept of homeopathy, when we become ill, it is *from within outwards*. Before disease-connected bacteria can grow uncontrolled within our bodies, there must be a disturbance to the vital force. As James Tyler Kent, one of the great American homeopaths, put it, "All true diseases of the economy flow from centre to circumference."

Apparent acute diseases that are actually brought about by diet, climate, environment, habits, stress, or physical trauma are not true diseases because they do not flow from the center outward; the initial disturbance is produced on the surface of the body and can be removed if the external cause is removed. Hahnemann believed that diseases entered the body in the form of *miasms*—subtle, imperceptible substances as immaterial as the vital force itself—that take hold of the vital force, causing it to express itself through the symptoms of its internal derangement. Interestingly, well before Pasteur, Koch, and others evolved the germ theory of disease toward the end of the nineteenth century, Hahnemann wrote of miasms as containing living organisms. In Hahnemann's time *miasm* generally meant an exhalation from a swampy area, which was believed to breed disease. During a cholera epidemic, Hahnemann wrote of the cholera miasm as a "swarm of those infinitely small, invisible, living organisms which are so hostile to human life and which most probably form the matter of cholera."[2] Although Hahnemann thus anticipated the modern concept of microbial infection, his writings clearly indicate that contagion cannot occur without prior susceptibility, i.e., derangement of the vital force. Modern homeopaths define a miasm as a blockage or a distortion of the normal flow of energy in the self-regulatory mechanism of the organism.

The true, or miasmatic, diseases, fall into two broad categories as follows:

1. *Acute diseases.* The acute disease, or acute miasm, is relatively short in duration and rapid in development, and it has a definite course, consisting of three phases: *(a)* a prodromal period, or onset; *(b)* a period of progress; and *(c)* a period of decline. All acute diseases, then, have a natural tendency to recovery—unless they are so severe as to terminate in the patient's death before the period of decline sets in. The vital force is generally capable of curing itself in the case of an acute disease, provided that the attack on the organism is not so violent as to produce death. In acute disease, homeopathy intervenes to relieve the sufferings of the patient, prevent his death, and speed his return to health.

2. *Chronic diseases.* In the case of what Hahnemann recognized as the chronic diseases, which are also miasmatic in character—that is, they flow into the body from the center outward—the course of the disease does not tend to recovery. There is again a prodromal period and a period of progress of the disease, but there is no period of decline. Under certain circumstances, as when the patient is relatively free from stress or when an acute disease supervenes, the chronic disease may quiet down and become virtually devoid of symptoms, but each time it is roused by adverse

2. From Samuel Hahnemann, *Lesser Writings*, quoted in G. Ruthven Mitchell, *Homeopathy* (London: W. H. Allen, 1975), p. 58.

conditions, the patient's chronic illness becomes worse than it was during the previous exacerbation.

Hahnemann believed that there would be no acute diseases without chronic diseases, that our predispositions to illness, or susceptibility to acute diseases, can be traced to the underlying chronic diseases that, over the millennia, have become the heritage of humankind.

Because the vital force does not have sufficient strength in and of itself to rid the organism of chronic disease, the patient can never be cured unless treated with the proper medicine, and even then, only insofar as irreversible tissue changes resulting from the chronic disease do not stand in the way. Homeopathy holds out the hope of a gentle, effective way of treating the chronic, or constitutional, diseases.

HOW MEDICINES WORK
The Law of Similars

The keystone of the homeopathic doctrine is the principle *similia similibus curantur* ("like shall be cured by like"). Hahnemann acknowledged that this principle was mentioned in the writings of Hippocrates, Paracelsus, and other empiricist predecessors (although it was not applied systematically by the earlier writers), but he got his first strong indications of the Law of Similars through direct experience, when, while attempting to determine what it was in the natural source of quinine that cured intermittent fever, he observed the ability of cinchona bark to produce the symptoms of intermittent fever in himself. As he proceeded to "prove" a number of other drugs, he observed that they too produced symptoms similar to those of the diseases in which they were curative. Going back through the medical literature, Hahnemann found other reported cases in which he deduced that the cure had been on the basis of similarity, although the physician reporting the cure was not necessarily aware of this principle. Hahnemann moved on to make the broad generalization that all disease is actively cured by the introduction of a second diseased state, similar to but stronger than the original disease. He found evidence of this idea not only in the historical reports of cures with drugs, but also in accidental cures in which a patient sick with a particular disease was cured of that disease when he became sick with another similar disease.

Of course it would be dangerous to attempt to cure a disease by introducing a more powerful natural disease into a sick patient, but Hahnemann had already shown that drugs were capable of producing artificial diseases within the human organism. Furthermore, he reasoned, artificial, drug-induced diseases were always stronger than natural diseases: not every healthy person exposed to a certain natural disease will develop the symptoms of that disease, whereas a drug in a sufficiently powerful dose will produce symptoms in any healthy person who takes it.

At the same time that he analyzed the medical literature for examples of (unconscious) homeopathic cures in the past, Hahnemann developed a large body of evidence related to the harmfulness of allopathic treatment. The drugs used by the allopaths were harmful in themselves, and the patients were debilitated by the methods used in "heroic medicine" —bleeding and purging and sweating; in addition, because allopathic medicines and procedures were directed against single symptoms or groups of symptoms rather than toward the patient as a whole, the patient was never truly cured. Hahnemann denounced the palliative and suppressive techniques of allopathy as injurious to the patient: a single symptom might be removed or suppressed, but the disease would go on unchecked, with perhaps a new drug disease added to it. Hahnemann thus formulated the Law of Similars.

Why should medicines act on this principle of similarity? Hahnemann offered two somewhat differing explanations. The first is that a disease is cured by another, similar but stronger, disease—whether the second disease is natural or drug-induced—by a process of displacement. In the course of provings of remedies, Hahnemann observed another phenomenon that also seemed to explain the curative action of similar drugs. When any drug is given to a healthy person, it produces two consecutive and opposite sets of symptoms, which Hahnemann termed the primary and secondary actions of the drug.

At first Hahnemann thought that both the primary and the secondary actions were true symptoms of the drug, but his eventual identification of the secondary action with the reactive power of the vital force led him to instruct provers to record only the primary actions of the drugs. Hahnemann provides an example:

After the profound stupefied sleep caused by opium (primary action) the following night will be all the more sleepless (reaction, secondary action). After the constipation produced by opium (primary action), diarrhea ensues (secondary action); and after purgation with medicines that irritate the bowels, constipation of several days' duration ensues (secondary action).[3]

When drugs are prescribed using the principle of similarity, the secondary action of the drug represents a rebound of the vital force. This rebound phenomenon can be observed in other areas of everyday life. If we stare at a red light, for example, when we take our eyes away from the light we see a green afterimage. This visual phenomenon is generated by our nervous system, without the physical presence of any green light in the "real world."

On the other hand, in nonhomeopathic treatment, the secondary action of a drug prescribed on the basis of dissimilarity will actually lead to a worsening of the patient's original condition.[4] Observing the effects of minor tranquilizers, we can see an example of this idea. The symptoms of anxiety, viewed as undesirable, may be temporarily suppressed, but after the drug has been somewhat metabolized, the symptoms often return with new vigor.

Thus, with the concept of primary and secondary symptoms, Hahnemann accounts for the operation of drugs on the principle of similarity and at the same time explains why palliative treatment is injurious to the patient.

We might note that the pattern of drug dependence seems to arise from this same mechanism. In order to counteract the effect of withdrawal (secondary action), from even a single dose of a drug, the individual takes another dose to reproduce the primary symptoms. This mechanism applies

3. Hahnemann, *Organon*, section 65.
4. Ibid., section 69.

not only in opiate and barbiturate addiction, but also in the habituation patterns that are induced by the frequent use of antacids, eye drops, nasal sprays, and the like.

Provings of Medicines

If the physician is to prescribe on the basis of the Law of Similars, he must have a knowledge of the symptoms produced by the various drugs at his disposal. These drug effects must be studied in healthy persons, for if the drugs are given to sick persons, the symptoms produced by the medicine are mixed up with the symptoms of the disease.[5]

Every medicine produces a different set of symptoms, just as all species of plants differ from one another in their structure and all mineral substances are different. In the case of highly toxic substances, very small doses must be administered to the prover. Milder drugs may be given in somewhat larger quantities; and in order to develop the full picture of the drug, the weakest drugs are best proved on subjects who are particularly sensitive.

In addition to being in good health, the prover must be conscientious and sufficiently intelligent to accurately report the drug effects. He must avoid all unusual disturbing influences while proving the drug, as well as all foods and drinks that will tend to have their own drug effect.[6] Before the commencement of the proving, the person conducting the experiment must take an inventory of the prover's state of health so that all preexisting symptoms in the prover can be

5. Although the concept of systematically proving drugs on healthy subjects is generally considered an innovation of Hahnemann's and was certainly popularized by the homeopaths, Hahnemann gives credit to the physician Albrecht von Haller for observing before him that this is the true method for determining the actions of drugs.

Another source of information about the disease-producing effects of drugs is the medical literature on poisonings. Hahnemann reviewed descriptions of cases of poisoning, both intentional and accidental, in which the effects of drugs were manifested very much in accord with his own observations in provings.

6. The prover should not cease his normal activities, however, or eliminate any normal habits or items of diet, since such changes in his patterns of living might produce symptoms of their own and thus confuse the picture of the drug effects.

subtracted from the sum of the effects that are observed after the administration of the drug. The drug is given either in a single dose, or, if it produces no effect, the dose may be repeated until symptoms appear. Once the prover has taken the first dose, all symptoms that are observed are to be interpreted as symptoms produced by the drug.

Each individual prover will develop only a relatively small number of symptoms, but a collection of the symptoms experienced by a large number of provers taking the same drug provides a full picture of the pathogenesis, or disease-producing effects, of the drug.

The prover is asked not only to record the symptoms he experiences, but to see how they are affected by various influences:

On experiencing any particular sensation from the medicine, it is useful, indeed necessary, in order to determine the exact character of the symptom, to assume various positions while it lasts, and to observe whether, by moving the part affected, by walking in the room or the open air, by standing, sitting or lying the symptom is increased, diminished or removed, and whether it returns on again assuming the position in which it was first observed,—whether it is altered by eating or drinking, or by any other condition, or by speaking, coughing, sneezing or any other action of the body, and at the same time to note at what time of the day or night it usually occurs in the most marked manner, whereby what is peculiar to and characteristic of each symptom will become apparent.[7]

Reactions of symptoms to external circumstances, whether drug symptoms or symptoms of natural diseases, are known as *modalities*. The modalities are important guides in characterizing the action of a drug, and similarly a patient's modalities in a diseased state may be important indicators of the proper drug for his condition. Such characterizations of symptoms as "worse on the right side, worse in the evening, better with motion, worse after eating" are examples of modalities.

Although it may appear illogical to assume that every twitch of the prover's eyelid, every twinge of pain, or every reaction to alteration in position or environment will be a true effect of the drug rather than mere coincidence, homeo-

7. Hahnemann, *Organon*, section 133.

paths have found that some of the most trivial symptoms appear again and again in the provings and play a prominent role in characterizing the action of a drug. Even an unusual symptom experienced by only one prover may be markedly characteristic of the drug. Homeopathic practice has shown that the selection of a remedy on the basis of one peculiar and characteristic symptom shared by a prover and a patient has led to many cures, thus validating not only the drug symptom but also the Law of Similars.

The Single Remedy

According to homeopathic doctrine, only a single remedy may be prescribed for the patient at any given time, for the simple and logical reason that only one drug is most similar to the symptoms presented by the patient. Furthermore, since the indications for prescribing are based on the provings of single substances, the only way that the action of such substances can be predicted is if they are prescribed singly, unmixed with other drugs. Allopathic practice may prescribe a number of drugs at the same time, each drug being aimed at a specific symptom or group of symptoms, and we have seen in recent years that such combining can lead to dangerous drug interactions.

Even in Hahnemann's day, when a relatively small number of substances had been proved, homeopaths found that the single most similar remedy would restore the patient to health. Today, with published provings of some two thousand substances, the homeopath can be even more confident that, with enough skill and patience, he will be able to find the *simillimum*—the remedy whose provings most closely match the symptoms presented by the patient.

Of course, homeopaths have also proved many chemical compounds, and many of the remedies from plant sources contain combinations of a number of different alkaloids and other chemicals. These complex substances, proved as discrete medicines, yield their own distinctive symptom images, which guide the practitioner in prescribing.

In principle, homeopaths would have no objection to compound remedies—consisting of more than one of the proved remedies—if these mixtures were proved as such. However, since we have no provings of such combinations, the practitioner must search for the *simillimum* among the single substances that have been properly proved.

Many homeopathic pharmaceutical manufacturers offer compound remedies for sale; however, such compound remedies represent a deviation from the strict Hahnemannian practice of homeopathy, and most classical prescribers today do not employ them.

HOW THE REMEDY IS SELECTED?

Homeopathy teaches that only by an accurate recording of all the patient's symptoms can the physician find the proper remedy for an illness, for it is through the symptoms that the vital force speaks and points to the remedy. Unlike orthodox medicine, which tends to concentrate on only those symptoms that fit conveniently into the doctor's idea of what disease the patient has, the homeopath accurately notes and records all symptoms, even if they appear unrelated to the patient's chief complaint. And it is often these accessory or concomitant symptoms that serve to individualize the patient and point to the correct remedy.

Taking the Case

Homeopathy, as we have seen, holds that it is only through the symptoms that the physician can know his patient's disease. Orthodox medicine attaches great significance to the results of "objective" laboratory tests, and the allopathic physician is guided in diagnosis and hence in treatment by these findings. Although modern homeopaths do attach more importance to pathologic laboratory tests than did their predecessors, such laboratory results cannot guide the homeopathic physician in prescribing, since the provings do not record these biochemical and pathological correlates of diseased states. In taking the case, the homeopath relies only on those things that are apparent to the senses, either through the verbal report of the patient and her attendants, or through direct observation of the patient. The homeopath operates on the assumption that all diseased states will be reflected in the patient's consciousness in the form of altered mental and emotional states, changes in sensation, or perceptible alterations in the function and appearance of parts of the body.

Homeopathy is thus dealing with extremely complex sources of information: the patients, with their failings of perception, their biases, their embarrassed reticence, their inattention to detail—all of it filtered through the medium of their own senses and reasoning as they receive information. It takes the highest freedom from prejudice and complete soundness of observation for the homeopath to record faithfully what he observes in the patient and not to be influenced by his own inclination to treat the disease before him with the same medication that "worked in Mrs. Jones's case" the week before.

The homeopath's initial interview with the patient may take one or two hours—in rather sharp contrast to the perfunctory fifteen-minute session in the orthodox specialist's examining room.

The first task is to record the patient's complaints in his own words. The homeopath employs slightly different strategies in taking the acute case versus the chronic case. In acute illness, the physician is interested only in all those things that have changed since the patient became ill; in the chronic case the physician will inquire about everything that has happened to the patient since birth. Chronic symptoms are frequently suppressed by acute illnesses, but if a patient manifests a chronic symptom while acutely ill, the physician attaches less importance to it than he does to the acute complaints. Once the acute illness is gone, the patient's chronic disease will be seen more clearly, and then it can be prescribed for. No matter whether the case is acute or chronic, the physician will place the greatest importance on the symptoms that the patient is manifesting, for it is only on the patient's present complaints that the homeopath can prescribe. Information about the patient's history may show how a chronic condition has developed and may point to a remedy that might be needed as the present symptoms regress.

The physician makes an accurate written record of all the

patient's symptoms, using the patient's own words. The provings are full of the common language of the provers as they reported their symptoms, and homeopaths find amazing correspondences between the expressions used by their patients and those recorded in the provings.

Then the physician elicits more specific information about each symptom the patient has reported, adding these details to the written record. If the patient has not volunteered information about bodily functions and, very importantly, about his mental state, the physician proceeds to inquire closely about these areas. The homeopath will also devote considerable attention to eliciting information about how the patient's symptoms are affected by external influences, such as heat, cold, eating, drinking, change of position, movement. The patient will be asked whether the symptoms are predominantly on one side of the body or the other and at what time of day they are worse. These details, known in homeopathy as *modalities*, are strongly marked in the symptom images of many of the remedies.

All these specific questions may strike us as trivial, but the physician, in constructing a picture of the patient's illness in these terms, is eliciting the very descriptions of symptoms that have been recorded in the provings of various drugs; it is often the seemingly inconsequential details that help in the selection of one among a number of possible remedies, all of which are more or less similar to the case, but only one of which bears a striking resemblance in these minute characteristic features as well.

After eliciting as much information as possible from a close questioning of the patient, the physician proceeds to note his own observations on the patient and then to determine whether these things were present in the patient in his healthy state. In homeopathy as in allopathy, the doctor's observations on the patient's mood, energy level, skin tone, breathing, and other details are components of a thorough routine physical examination. Contemporary homeopaths stress the importance of a complete physical examination, but the homeopath attaches equal importance to the patient's subjective sensations, his mental state, everything that characterizes the patient as a whole, and as an individual.

It is also important for the physician to take into consideration the patient's disposition—whether he is overly sensitive or hypochondriacal, or whether he exaggerates his symptoms in order to get faster relief. The importance of the symptoms must be weighed in light of such observations. The patient's tendency to exaggerate or to minimize his symptoms is considered an important symptom in itself.

Now is the first instance in the therapeutic process where the patient may derive genuine placebo benefit from the homeopathic method. There is probably a good deal of intrinsic therapeutic value in the homeopath's devoting so much time and attention to every trivial detail of the patient's illness, style of life, and mental state. A patient questioned so closely must feel somewhat reassured that the doctor is taking a genuine interest in her and will do everything possible to help restore her health.

The taking of a case in homeopathy may have a certain educational benefit as well. When the patient learns to recognize that derangements of her internal state of health are reflected in her consciousness, she may, if as her treatment progresses she continues to monitor her internal state, actually learn to reach the healing powers of the vital force, much as yogis learn to control the "involuntary" processes in their bodies, and as patients given biofeedback training learn to control their blood pressure, tension headaches, and acid secretions that aggravate ulcerative conditions.

Classifying the Symptoms

In order to evaluate the symptom picture he now has before him, the physician must classify the symptoms according to their importance and the degree to which they are marked in the patient. There are three classes of symptoms: (1) general, (2) common, and (3) particular.

The *common symptoms* are those that appear in many cases of disease—such as fever, nausea, or headache—and also those that appear in most cases of a certain type of disease, such as rash in measles. It is often these symptoms that will bring the patient to the doctor's office, but they are the least important when it comes to selecting a remedy, since many remedies share these symptoms in common. Here again is where homeopathy deviates from orthodox practice, for when the allopathic doctor can identify a group of symptoms as "belonging to" a certain "disease entity," he will treat on the basis of the common symptoms alone, disregarding any individual peculiarities that the patient may present in his particular case of measles or flu or pneumonia.

The *general symptoms* are considered by the homeopath first in importance. They are the symptoms that tell how the patient feels in himself, as a whole. Mental symptoms fall into this category and are among the most important, since the patient's mental state is a strong reflection of his overall feeling of illness or well-being. Some homeopathic prescribers are guided in their selection of a remedy by the mentals alone, using the other symptoms simply for confirmation of their choice of a remedy.

The *particular symptoms* are those that pertain to any given organ, and to the homeopath they are not as significant in the process of selecting a remedy as are the generals. However, there may be a thread that runs through a number of symptoms: the patient may have an earache in the right ear, pain in the right side of the abdomen, and numbness of the right arm. The modality of location running through a number of particular symptoms itself becomes a general symptom. Qualities that are ascribed to any given organ are particulars; but *if the same quality or attribute is ascribed to a number of organs, it becomes a general symptom.* Thus, modalities—such as amelioration or aggravation from motion, from heat or cold, from eating or drinking, from change in weather or change in position—are often general symptoms.

In order to arrive at a truly individualized, characteristic picture of the patient, the homeopathic physician looks for those strange, rare, and peculiar symptoms that set one case apart from all other superficially similar cases. Such strange, rare, and peculiar symptoms may be unusual in themselves. For example, characteristic of the remedy *Thuja* is the patient's fixed idea that she is very delicate, that she is made of glass, and that she will break. Or, the symptom may be strange because it is contrary to what one would expect, such as the ignatia symptom of inflamed, throbbing, hot body parts that are not painful when handled and are often ameliorated by pressure. Strange, rare, and peculiar symptoms may be generals (including mentals) or particulars; by their very nature they can never be commons, and they are generally given more weight than other symptoms of the same class.

Finally, all symptoms must be graded. Each class of symptoms—the general, the common, and the particular—are assigned first, second, or third grade, according to the degree to which they are marked, the first grade being the most marked. Similarly, the symptoms of the remedies have been graded according to the incidence of their appearance among provers: those that appear in the majority of provers are of the first grade, those that are seen in a few provers are second grade, and those that occur in only an isolated case or two—but are still sufficiently marked to qualify as genuine symptoms—are assigned the third grade.

This classifying and grading of symptoms helps the homeopath to assign relative weights to the patient's complaints, just as the symptoms are weighted in the provings of the remedies, so that the most accurate match can be made between the picture of the patient and that of the proper remedy.

Selecting the *Simillimum*

Once the symptoms have been analyzed, the physician is ready to search for the *simillimum*, the most similar remedy. His tools for this task, in addition to his own clinical experience and his personal familiarity with the symptom images of a large number of drugs, consist of two sorts of reference books—the *materia medica* and the *repertory*, some of which are listed in Appendix A. For each remedy that has been proved, the materia medica contains a listing of the symptoms that have been elicited in the provers following the administration of that drug. Some remedies have not been completely proved, and so the symptom images are not complete. Additional information on drug symptoms is derived from toxicological reports of the effects of poisoning by each of the drugs in overdose and from clinical experience that confirms that a given remedy has been successful in eradicating a given symptom.

Under each of the remedies in the materia medica, the symptoms are arranged under generals, mentals, parts of the body, modalities, etc. The physician cannot read through the 2,000-odd drug pictures in a comprehensive materia medica each time he wants to select a remedy for a particular case, so he makes use of a second type of book, a repertory, which serves as an index to symptoms. In the repertory, symptoms are listed under headings, or *rubrics*, such as mentals, parts of the body, etc.; the individual symptoms, and each of the things that modifies them, are followed by a list of all the drugs that have produced that particular symptom or that particular modality for a symptom. To aid the physician in recognizing the more strongly marked symptoms of a drug, or the more characteristic drugs for a symptom, in some repertories, the drugs producing the symptom in the first grade are printed in bold face, those of the second grade are in italics, and those of the third grade are in normal type.

The job of the physician, then, is to write down after each of the patient's symptoms, or after each of several selected symptoms, all the drugs he finds in the repertory associated with that symptom. After he has gone through the patient's symptoms in this manner, certain remedies will stand out as running through a large number of symptoms. At this point, if the doctor has taken the case completely enough, only a few drugs will be prominently repeated in the repertorization. When the physician then turns to the materia medica and reads the complete symptom picture for each of these few drugs, one of them should stand out as the *simillimum*.

The process of repertorization is as tedious and time-consuming as it sounds. As the homeopathic practitioner, through his practice, becomes familiar with more and more of the remedies and their action in his patients, he is apt to recognize the images of certain medicines in many of his cases, as if he were recognizing an old friend. Still, he will consult the repertory and the materia medica to confirm his perceptions.

It has been the habit of some homeopaths to prescribe on the basis of *keynotes*—listings of the most characteristic and peculiar symptoms associated with each remedy. Repertorizing by keynotes alone would obviously be a lot simpler than going through all the patient's symptoms and repertorizing each one of them, but the most successful homeopaths warn that there is no shortcut to prescribing, just as there is no shortcut to the examination of the patient.

Another possible way of bypassing the time-consuming process of repertorization is through the use of the computer. Chapter 5 contains a brief discussion of a project that is under way in the United States to assess the value of such an approach.

The *Remedy Epidemicus*

As we have indicated, the homeopath carefully selects a remedy on the basis of the totality of the patient's symptoms, treating the patient as a distinct individual unlike any other patient he has seen. Although this principle is always implicit in the homeopath's case taking and treatment, we should note that his choices of a remedy are narrowed considerably in the instance of epidemic diseases that attack large segments of the population over a relatively short period of time. In such epidemics, the homeopath carefully examines the first few cases that come to him and generally finds that one remedy, or a small number of remedies, covers the symptoms produced by the disease in all the individuals he examines. The symptomatology of an acute epidemic disease is so strongly marked that it will effectively suppress a patient's underlying constitutional symptomatology; thus, individualization is not so prominent a concern. The remedy determined to be the *simillimum* in an epidemic disease is known as the *remedy epidemicus*, and the conscientious homeopath will immediately communicate his determinations to fellow practitioners in his area so that they can benefit from his case taking and keep this remedy (or remedies) in mind as they are called on to treat cases of the epidemic disease.

Among Hahnemann's more striking successes in his early years of homeopathic practice was his use of *belladonna* in a scarlet fever epidemic. Quite by accident, Hahnemann found that *belladonna* not only cured his scarlet fever patients on the basis of the Law of Similars, but also that it acted as a preventative. One of the families he was treating had several children, one of whom had been given *belladonna* for another problem entirely, and of all the children in the family, this child was the only one not to come down with the disease. Even in allopathic practice, Hahnemann's example led many physicians to use *belladonna* both as a cure and as a prophylactic in epidemics of scarlet fever.

HOW THE MEDICINES ARE PREPARED

One common area of confusion about the meaning of homeopathy is the belief that homeopathy uses herbal remedies. Vegetable substances, including many medicinal herbs, have been a source of homeopathic remedies since Hahnemann's time, but homeopathy makes equal use of substances from the mineral and animal kingdoms—including many substances that in their natural state are both virulent poisons and biologically inert. It is only by means of the special way in which such remedies are prepared for homeopathic use that they are thought to acquire their medicinal powers.

Sources of Remedies

The homeopathic pharmacopoeia defines the vegetable, mineral, animal, or other source for each of the homeopathic remedies. Because the provings record the effects of remedies that have been derived from specific sources (for example, a particular variety of a certain species of plant growing in a specific location), all remedies should be prepared from identical sources, in order that their effects will be identical.[8]

---

8. A recent book by James Stephenson, M.D. (see Appendix A), gives instructions on preparing your own remedies from plants in your garden and from common household or drugstore items. Although his attempt to make homeopathic medicines accessible is admirable, we might raise some serious questions about whether the individual is indeed using a proved remedy in such a case. There is also the serious possibility that in the process of preparing the remedy, the experimenter may at the same time be bringing out the medicinal effects of other unknown substances that may have come into contact with these vegetable sources—insecticides, animal excreta, and the like.

The Minimum Dose

When Hahnemann began prescribing on the basis of the Law of Similars, he used the large doses employed in the orthodox medicine of his time. However, when the remedy selected was homeopathic to the case (that is, when its action in the sick person demonstrated that it was correctly chosen on the basis of similarity), he noted that his patient would experience a severe aggravation of symptoms through the primary (or similar) action of the drug. Hahnemann began experimenting with reduced dosages, and he observed that, in sufficiently small quantities, the remedy would not produce a serious aggravation of the symptoms but would still effect a cure through its stimulation of the reactive power of the vital force (secondary symptoms). As a result of this experimentation, it came to be an accepted principle of homeopathy that the proper dose of a medicine is the minimum amount that is required to effect a cure; that is, the minimum amount that will stimulate the vital force to react against the disease and bring about a state of health. In practical terms, the proper dose could be defined as the minimum amount needed to produce a slight aggravation of the symptoms.

Potentized Remedies

Hahnemann's earliest experiments with reduction of the dose consisted of a simple dilution of the original drug to a high level of attenuation. There was a point where the diluted substance would no longer exert a medicinal effect, and it was then that Hahnemann discovered a revolutionary approach to the preparation of medicines—the concept of *dynamization* or *potentization*.

Starting with a crude substance or a tincture, the original medicinal substance was subjected to a process of serial dilution, with each step of dilution accompanied by a vigorous shaking, or *succussion*. Hahnemann found that progressive succussed dilutions of the medicine acquired increased curative power, at the same time reducing the likelihood of undesirable aggravation of the patient's symptoms. The

process of serial dilution and succussion is known in homeopathy as potentization: the higher the potency, the lower the
concentration of the original medicinal substance.

If the original substance was insoluble in water or alcohol
(which Hahnemann assumed were medicinally inert and could
therefore be used as solvents), it was *triturated*, i.e., reduced
to a powder in mortar and pestle, with ninety-nine parts
of milk sugar (also assumed to be medicinally inert), to one
part of the original medicine.[9] Trituration is a painstaking
process requiring about one hour for each dilution of 1:100.
After the initial 1:100 trituration—called the *first centesimal
dilution*—has been prepared, one part of this mixture is
triturated with a further 99 parts of milk sugar by the same
process, yielding a 1:10,000 mixture of the original substance, or the *second centesimal dilution*. The process is
repeated a third time to produce the *third centesimal dilution*, or one part of the medicine to one million parts of milk
sugar. Hahnemann observed that at this point the powder
would be "soluble" in water or alcohol, and further serial
dilutions would be prepared by adding one part of the mixture to 99 parts of water or alcohol, each time increasing the
dilution by a factor of 100.[10]

If the original substance is soluble in alcohol, the starting
point is a *tincture*, a concentrated alcohol solution, which is
then used to make a 1:99 solution. With each successive
liquid dilution, the mixture is subjected to a series of sharp
succussions, or shakes, which Hahnemann and homeopaths
after him believed brought out hidden medicinal qualities of
the drug. For this purpose Hahnemann rapped the container
against a felt pad, using the heel of his hand to protect the

9. We may question Hahnemann's assumption that alcohol and milk
sugar are inert. Certainly the drug effects of alcohol in measurable doses
are quite marked; and many people suffer from a "milk allergy," or
lactose deficiency, that renders them unable to tolerate milk sugar in
the diet. At any rate, if alcohol and milk sugar do acquire a medicinal
effect through the process of potentization, their effects are a constant,
superadded to the pathogenesis of *all* the homeopathic remedies and in-
distinguishable from the symptom images of the remedies themselves.

10. In his use of "solutions" of triturations, Hahnemann anticipated
the science of colloid chemistry, or the dispersion of insoluble substances
in a liquid medium.

glass from breaking. In the laboratories of modern homeo-pathic pharmaceutical manufacturers, this tedious process has become mechanized to some extent, but long trituration and repeated succussion are still critical elements in the dilution process.

While the *centesimal scale of dilution* (1:100) is the most widely used in the United States today, other systems are also used. In the *decimal scale*, each successive dilution is in the ratio of 1:10 rather than 1:100. *Centesimal potencies* are expressed as 1c, or simply 1, for the *first centesimal* (1:100); 2c or 2 for the second centesimal (1:10,000); and so on. *Decimal potencies* are expressed as 1x (1:10); 2x (1:100); etc.[11]

Among the most common potencies used are the 3rd, 6th, 12th, and 30th. All of these are available over the counter in homeopathic pharmacies in the United States, but the higher potencies are reserved for professionals. This restriction on the dispensing of the higher potencies underlines the para-doxical claim that the very highest potencies have the most power to stir up the reactive vital force and should therefore not be placed in inexpert hands.

Avogadro's Law and the Ultramolecular Dose

When Hahnemann began treating his patients with high dilutions of homeopathic remedies, his critics immediately argued that such high potencies could not possibly have any medicinal effect because of the extreme attenuation of the medicinal substance. In 1811, the Italian physicist Amadeo Avogadro published a paper demonstrating that one gram mole of any compound or element (its molecular weight expressed in grams) contained approximately 6×10^{23} mole-cules. Therefore, in any given weight of a substance that can be broken down into molecules, the number of molecules can be known if the weight is known. If this quantity is then

11. Other systems for preparation of potencies have also been used. The sixth and last edition of the *Organon* gives instructions for what is known as the fiftieth milesimal scale, which increases the dilution in each successive phase by a ratio of 1:50,000!

subjected to serial dilution, there will be a point where none of the original substance is likely to remain in a given sample of the dilution.

Let us assume that we start with one gram mole of the original substance—for example, sodium chloride, whose molecular weight is 48.46 grams. Each of the original 48.46 grams of sodium chloride contain 6×10^{23} molecules. To this amount of sodium chloride we add 99 parts of water and then take a hundredth part of this solution. This hundredth part will contain $\frac{1}{100}$ of the original number of molecules, or $$\frac{6 \times 10^{23}}{10^2} = 6 \times 10^{21} \text{ molecules.}$$ To this we add 99 parts of water, and again take a hundredth part, resulting in 6×10^{19} molecules of the original substance (assuming always that the solution is evenly mixed throughout). And so we progress with this process until a point where the remaining molecules are expressed as 6×10^1. At this point, if we take a hundredth part of the solution, the remaining molecules will be expressed as 6×10^{-1}, or $\frac{6}{10}$. A molecule cannot be divided, so far as we know, by merely mechanical means, so from this point on such mathematical expressions are merely statements of a declining probability that a single molecule of the original substance will be present in any sample of this level of dilution!

Hahnemann was not blind to the apparent paradox of a substance increasing in medicinal power as its quantity decreased—even to the point of being physically absent from the solution. He believed that the process of dilution and succussion actually released a "spiritlike power" that was particularly adapted to work on the equally spiritlike vital force in man.

How can homeopathically prepared remedies acquire this "spiritlike power"? In recent years, a number of laboratory experiments have been performed by homeopaths to investigate the activity of high potencies. Even Hahnemann had an intimation of the highly attenuated forms of energy—such as electromagnetic radiation or subatomic particles—that modern science has unveiled. Using the analogy of the magnet,

Hahnemann speaks of the communication of a dynamic force from one substance to another:

It is not in the corporeal atoms of these highly dynamized medicines, nor their physical or mathematical surfaces . . . that the medicinal energy is found. More likely, there lies invisible in the moistened globule or in its solution, an unveiled, liberated, specific, medicinal force contained in the medicinal substance which acts dynamically by contact with the living animal fibre upon the whole organism (without communicating to it anything material however highly attenuated) and acts more strongly the more free and more immaterial the energy has become through the dynamization.[12]

Some modern attempts to account for the activity of the high potencies will be found in chapter 5. Regardless of the scientific explanations advanced, however, homeopaths today speak of the high potencies as transmitting a pattern, rather than exerting a gross drug effect. With the vast number of drugs to choose from, homeopaths reason that the *simillimum* will fit the patient on a dynamic plane, acting as a template to provide an energy pattern by means of which the disordered vital force can readjust itself.

Improbable as the activity of the high potencies may appear to common sense, homeopaths offer the evidence of 170 years of experience to attest to the powers of potentized remedies. Such evidence lies both in the provings of the high potencies and in actual clinical experience. In the treatment of chronic diseases, homeopaths claim that their patients may experience extremely disturbing effects from the use of the high potencies of a properly selected drug. Troublesome old symptoms that the patient may have entirely forgotten may reappear during the course of constitutional treatment with very high potencies. Subjects in provings similarly describe skin eruptions, aches and pains, and altered mental states following the administration of high potencies of homeopathic remedies.

Hahnemann's work with the infinitesimal dose led to a further discovery. Many substances that were biologically inert in their crude form developed marked medicinal pow-

12. Hahnemann, *Organon*, note to section 11.

ers when subjected to trituration or serial dilution and succussion. Hahnemann used elemental gold, biologically inert
in the crude state, for the treatment of suicidal tendencies.
Certain vegetable substances, such as the spores of the club
moss, *Lycopodium*, that were generally thought to have no
medicinal effects in the crude state, have become some of
the most important and powerful of the homeopath's armamentarium of medicines.

Similarly, many substances that are highly toxic in the
crude state—for example, arsenic, strychnine, and snake
venom—may be used as medicines when sufficiently diluted
and are believed to be very powerful in high potencies.

Hahnemann's principle of the minimum dose, as well as
his observations on the power of the vital force to rebound
and produce secondary symptoms, anticipates the *Arndt-
Schulz law*, an allopathic rule formulated toward the end of
the nineteenth century: "Weak stimuli increase physiologic
activity and very strong stimuli inhibit or abolish activity"
or, "Small drug doses kindle vital activities, moderate doses
increase them, large doses depress them, and largest doses
remove them." This "allopathic homeopathic principle" reaf-
firmed Hahnemann's observation that substances that can
kill in large quantities can stimulate and cure in small doses.

Since Avogadro's law implies that, beyond the 24th decimal (or the 12th centesimal) dilution there will remain no
molecules of the original substance, potencies above the
24th decimal dilution are considered *ultramolecular* doses.
Potencies such as the 3rd, 6th, and 12th are considered *low
potencies*; the 30th and 200th are commonly employed as
medium potencies; and those above the 200th are called
high potencies. The high potencies are frequently prescribed in the treatment of acute and chronic diseases, and
according to the reports of homeopathic prescribers, the
results are often spectacular.

The principle of potentization has always been a controversial subject for homeopathy. It has been one of the objects
of greatest derision among opponents of the homeopathic
doctrine, and it has produced sharp division even among the
ranks of homeopaths. When homeopathy was at its most

popular in the United States, many homeopaths were using only tinctures or low potencies, and even today some practitioners prefer to avoid the higher potency range. As long as they are prescribing on the basis of the Law of Similars and using remedies prepared according to Hahnemann's instructions, such homeopaths are still practicing homeopathy in the classical sense, for the use of high potencies is not an essential element of the homeopathic doctrine. Today, however, when cases require it, homeopaths will generally use the whole range of potencies, from crude drugs or tinctures all the way through the hundred thousandth (CM) or higher, depending on the requirements of the individual case, and always prescribing on the basis of the Law of Similars.

Some of the most prominent homeopathic physicians have had their personal struggles with the concept of potentization, as the following passage from James Tyler Kent's *Lectures on Homeopathic Philosophy* will illustrate:

I remember when I first read from Hahnemann that potentized medicines would cure the sick that it seemed to me a mystery. I had no knowledge upon which to found belief in such things. I began to carry out the law, but with these means I was able to cure only superficial complaints. My work was far from satisfactory, yet it was somewhat better than the old things, it was milder than physicking and purging and emesis. Of course I rested upon my opinions and belief for my knowledge; everyone does that.

Later I resolved to test the 30th potency to see if there was not yet medicine in it, and I prepared with my own hands the 30th potency of Podophyllum with water on the centesimal scale, after the fashion of Hahnemann. . . . This was during an epidemic of diarrhoea that looked like Podophyllum, but I had not the courage to give the 30th and still continued to use my stronger medicines. One day a child was brought into my office in the mother's arms. She brought it in hastily, and it did not seem as if it could live long. It was an infant, and while it lay in her arms a thin yellowish fecal stool ran over my carpet. The odor struck me as. like that I had been reading about as the odor of the Podophyllum stool; it was horribly offensive, stinking, and the stool was so copious that the mother made the remark that she did not know where it all came from. I said to myself, this is a case upon which to test Hahnemann's 30th potency. So I fixed up some of the Podophyllum 30 and put it on the child's tongue, and sent the mother home, fearing that the child would soon die, as it was very ill, face pinched and drawn, cadaveric, and had a dreadful odor about it. Next morning when making my rounds I had to pass the house. I expected to see crepe on the door. I did not dare to call, though I was very much worried about it, so I drove past, but there was no crepe on the door. I drove home again that way, although it was quite a distance out of the way, and still there was no crepe on the door; but standing in the doorway was the grandmother, who said; "Doctor, the baby is all right this morning." Then I began to feel better, thinking I had not killed it. Perhaps some of you have been in the same state of mind.

That little child did not need any more medicine. After that I had quite a number of Podophyllum cases, and the 30th did the work to my astonishment. It was different from anything I had ever seen; the cures were almost instantaneous, it seemed as if there would be no more stool after the first dose of medicine. I did not always give the single dose. I used the 30th all the season, and then made up my mind that if the 30th of Podophyllum was good other 30ths would also be, and I ought to have as many of them as possible. I made a good many 30ths by hand, and finally succeeded in making up one hundred and twenty-six remedies, some of them in the 200th potency, and these I used. Then I procured a set of 200ths and higher and practiced with them. I followed on in this way and in a few years I discovered that by giving higher and higher potencies the remedies seemed to operate more and more interiorly.[13]

Forms of Homeopathic Remedies

Homeopathic remedies are available in several forms: (1) mother tinctures, (2) triturations, (3) tablets or pillules, and (4) globules.

Mother tinctures are alcohol extracts of the original substance. They are generally used for external application or for the preparation of potencies, though tinctures are sometimes given internally as well.

Triturations are powders, or tablets made of powder, consisting of the original substance ground up (as described earlier) with a quantity of milk sugar. They may be placed directly on the tongue or added to distilled water for administration to the patient.

13. James Tyler Kent, M.D., *Lectures on Homeopathic Philosophy* (New Delhi: B. Jain Publishers, 1974), pp. 97–99.

Tablets (or pillules) are sugar tablets, generally of 1 to 1¼ grain size, upon which have been placed a few drops of the liquid potency of the remedy. They may be taken dry on the tongue or dissolved in distilled water. The pillules are considered very stable and will keep indefinitely if they are stored in an airtight container, away from other substances that might contaminate them, and not exposed to excessive heat or sunlight.

Globules are sugar tablets about the size of poppy seeds (their size having been the occasion of considerable ridicule among opponents of homeopathy), and they are prepared and administered in the same manner as the tablets.

When it was introduced by Hahnemann, the use of sugar as a base for homeopathic medicines was a novel idea. Most of the medicines of the time consisted of vile-tasting concoctions or equally offensive chemical compounds, and they were administered without any attempt to mask their taste and generally in large quantities. The use of sugar as a vehicle for the administration of medicines was one of the innovations in homeopathy that was subsequently taken over by orthodox medicine. Homeopathy, however, has not taken the next step that has been taken by the manufacturers of allopathic drugs: colored tablets are not used, on the principle that the coloring matter may have a drug effect in itself. We have seen in recent years that the suspicions of the homeopaths were well founded, as problems such as the hyperkinetic syndrome in children are being associated with the use of dyes in foodstuffs.

THE FIRST PRESCRIPTION
Potency Selection

After determining the remedy that is most similar to the patient's total symptom picture, the homeopath has the further task of selecting the proper potency of the indicated remedy. Unlike the selection of the remedy, the choice of potency is not governed by hard-and-fast rules; thus, potency selection might be considered part of the "art" of homeopathy.

Hahnemann generally restricted his potency range to the 30th and lower. The highest potency he had in his collection of remedies was reportedly 200th, and he states in the *Organon* that no potency higher than the 30th should be needed in the treatment of illness. Contemporary homeopathic experience tends to contradict Hahnemann's claim, for many homeopaths today are regularly prescribing the high potencies—the 10,000th, the 100,000th, and upward. It is possible that these higher potencies are needed because of the more sophisticated suppressive effects of modern drugs; perhaps chronic conditions have been driven farther inward and cannot be reached by a potency that approaches the material plane. The contamination of our environment by trace quantities of toxic substances, background radiation, and the like may have an additional effect on our response to homeopathic remedies. Some homeopaths, however, adhere strictly to the Law of Similars and still restrict their prescribing to the lower end of the potency range.

The selected remedy, in order to be a true *simillimum*, must match not only the patient's symptoms but also the dynamic plane of the disease at the time the patient presents himself for treatment. Because the mental sphere of the human organism is innermost, approaching the immateriality of the vital force itself, the high potencies are reported to produce the best results in cases with predominantly mental symptoms. Homeopaths who employ the whole range of potencies may treat mental illnesses and problems of psychic origin with the 10,000th and upward. Where the illness is organic—that is, where the symptoms consist of tissue change and other problems on the material plane—the lower or medium potencies are more suitable. In general, where there is deep, serious physical pathology, potency selection is restricted to the 200th and lower, since higher potencies might stir up the reactive vital force more than the patient can tolerate. Similarly, in older people with reduced vitality, prescribers do not go above the 200th.

Children are reported to respond especially well to high potencies, partly because most of their troubles are acute in nature and their symptoms clear-cut. In children with deep, chronic pathology, however, prescribing is again limited to the 200th and lower.

Some patients are sensitive to any remedy they are given; such people often demonstrate a generalized nervousness and a sensitivity to everything—including their surroundings, as well as other people. In such patients, and in patients who have idiosyncrasies to certain remedies, the medium- or low-potency range is employed.

Sometimes the homeopathic practitioner will not feel that he has sufficient symptomatology for a remedy to be absolutely indicated. In such cases, he will begin with a potency in the middle range, such as the 30th or 200th; in unclear cases where there is also deep pathology present, he will prescribe as low as the 6th or the 12th.

The rationale underlying the selection of potencies is that the crude drug, or the tincture, will produce an effect on virtually anyone; as the stages of dilution progress toward the higher potencies, the patient must have an increasing susceptibility to the remedy in order for it to act. In other words, the highest potencies will produce an effect only in those patients whose symptom pictures closely match the symptom picture for the remedy. George Vithoulkas, the great homeopath, refers to this matching on the deepest dynamic plane as a sort of "resonance" between the energy field of the patient's vital force and the energy field of the potentized remedy; at the higher levels of potentization, the remedy is no longer acting on a material level, just as in deep psychic and functional disturbances the forces involved are not on the physical plane.

Some cases are incurable, with advanced pathological changes, and are open only to palliation. The lower or medium potencies are used here, and when the *simillimum* happens to be a deep-acting remedy, prescribers will often avoid it entirely, prescribing a related, only partially similar remedy in a low or medium potency to afford palliation without stirring up the reactive forces of the organism.

Just as too-frequent repetition of a remedy may produce an inadvertent proving, so may repetition of the same potency implant in the patient a chronic drug disease. When a given potency of a remedy has exhausted its action, a high potency is often reported to continue the curative process. Thus homeopathic prescribers will often run through the whole range of potencies to the highest available and then return to the original potency prescribed to be sure that the remedy has done all it can. Of course, this process is only applied as long as the patient continues to present the same symptoms; once the symptoms change, the case must be retaken and a new *simillimum* found.

The Single Dose

We have seen that a single remedy is selected on the basis of its similarity to the patient's symptoms. The remedy is given to the patient in a single dose. The meaning of the single dose is open to interpretation: some homeopaths will administer the remedy in divided doses in a high potency at short intervals; others will give one potency to start and then a higher or lower one some hours later. Another variation on the idea of the single dose is known as *plussing*, in which the dose is dissolved in water, two teaspoonfuls are taken, and most of the rest discarded. More water is then added, up to the original amount of liquid, and the solution is stirred (to provide succussion); two teaspoonfuls are taken as a second dose, and the process is repeated for each successive dose. The purpose of plussing is to give the same remedy in a slightly different, higher potency in each successive dose.

On the whole, though, we can consider any of the methods described above as a single dose; for practical purposes, let us assume that the remedy is given in a single, undivided dose. The important thing for the prescriber to bear in mind after administering the first dose is not to repeat the dose, but to watch and wait. Each remedy has its own rhythm, manifesting its symptoms in a characteristic order and at a characteristic pace, and to give another dose at this point might break up the rhythm of a remedy that has already begun to work. The homeopathic prescriber must have the greatest patience, simply observing the patient to see if the remedy is working. An absolute rule in homeopathy is that when favorable reaction sets in, the administration of the remedy must stop.

Once reaction has occurred, the remedy has taken hold of the vital force and must be allowed to expend itself according to its own characteristic rhythm. In acute diseases, homeopaths say that favorable reaction may set in within a few minutes to a few hours; in chronic diseases, because the pace of their development is slower, reaction will similarly be slower, perhaps a few days to a few weeks. The remedies themselves also differ in the speed with which their action is exhausted; the interaction of a fast- and short-acting acute remedy with the fast-progressing acute disease may call for a repetition of the remedy at short intervals, whereas the chronic remedy may hold for months, years, or even a lifetime.

WATCHING THE CASE
Hering's Law

After the prescription has been given, the homeopath must wait and watch. The patient's reaction will indicate whether the remedy has been correct or not. But, in following the case, the homeopath has more to go on than merely the patient's sense of improvement in his well-being. When a patient is treated according to homeopathic rules, experience has shown that symptoms appear and disappear in a definite order. Constantine Hering (1800–1880), known as the father of American homeopathy, provided a set of guidelines that assist the physician in determining the progress and prognosis of a case. According to *Hering's law* (the most important addition to Hahnemann's original formulation of the homeopathic doctrine), symptoms disappear *from within outward, from above downward, from more important to less important organs, and in the reverse order of their appearance.* That is, the remedy acts first by taking hold of the innermost part of the human economy, and the symptoms leave the innermost, or more vital organs, moving from the interior to the exterior of the body; also, first from the head, then from the torso, and last from the extremities. As we shall see, Hahnemann's theory traces many serious chronic conditions to earlier suppressions of less serious surface symptoms, such as skin eruptions. In the course of the homeopathic cure, the older symptoms may reappear after the symptoms affecting vital organs have passed off. When cure takes place in this order, the homeopath knows that it is proceeding in the correct manner, and that the remedy selected was appropriate. Hering's law is not entirely unknown outside the realm of homeopathy. It is equally applied in naturopathy, for example, as a means of assessing the progress of a case under treatment.

We might ask how the homeopath determines whether the case is actually progressing in the correct direction. To deal with this question, George Vithoulkas proposes a three-dimensional model of the human organism, in the shape of a cone, in which the mental, emotional, and physical planes are represented respectively by an inner, middle, and outer concentric cone. Along each of these cones, various organs or functions are arranged, with the most vital at the tip of the cone and the least vital at the base. Thus, in the course of the progress of a case, symptoms may move either outward, from the center toward the periphery (from mental to emotional to physical), or they may move downward on the same plane, for example the physical, through a descending hierarchy of physical organs. This model helps to visualize the concept that the mental part of man represents his most important, innermost level of functioning. Indeed, Vithoulkas observes that the best measure of whether a patient is getting better is whether he feels better within himself—whether he is happy and creative—regardless of how much physical discomfort he may be feeling. Still, it can be difficult for the homeopath to evaluate the actual direction the symptoms are taking; for example, if a state of extreme anxiety recedes and is replaced by a spinal cord lesion, are the symptoms proceeding in the proper direction or not?

Vithoulkas's model cannot answer all such questions with certainty, but the necessity of having some sort of model for purposes of reference becomes clear when we attempt to apply Hering's law in practice.

The Homeopathic Aggravation

As we have stated, Hahnemann began prescribing on the basis of the Law of Similars, using doses equivalent to those employed in allopathic practice and later reducing the dose in order to avoid the homeopathic aggravations he observed when the *simillimum* added its own, similar symptoms to those for which the patient was being treated. Even with potentized doses, it is not unusual for the patient to experience a slight aggravation of his symptoms shortly after administration of the remedy:

But though it is certain that a homeopathically selected remedy does, by reason of its appropriateness and the minuteness of the dose, gently remove and annihilate the acute disease analogous to it, without manifesting its other unhomeopathic symptoms, that is to say, without the production of new, serious disturbances, yet it usually, immediately after ingestion—for the first hour, or for a few hours—causes a kind of slight aggravation when the dose has not been sufficiently small and (where the dose has been somewhat too large, however, for a considerable number of hours) which has so much resemblance to the original disease that it seems to the patient to be an aggravation of his own disease. But it is, in reality, nothing more than an extremely similar *medicinal disease*, somewhat exceeding in strength the original affection.[14]

Such a slight aggravation of the patient's symptoms is taken as a favorable sign and should be followed by an improvement in his condition.

To illustrate how the homeopath watches his case after administering the remedy, let us look at twelve possible outcomes listed by Kent. These do not necessarily exhaust the possibilities, and they have been combined and arranged in different ways by later homeopathic practitioners, but Kent's twelve situations—with Kent's interpretations and a few additional ones by later prescribers—will give us a chance to see how the homeopath applies Hering's law, how he recognizes incurable cases, how he uses the higher and lower potencies, and how he can tell if the remedy is actually mixing up the case or making it worse.

14. Hahnemann, *Organon*, section 157.

1. *Prolonged aggravation with subsequent decline of the patient.* In this case, the remedy prescribed has gone too deep; it has stirred up the vital force in a patient who is gravely ill, as in a patient who has far-advanced pathological tissue changes but sufficient vitality to produce symptoms. Or, the case is incurable, and vital reaction to the remedy was not possible. In such incurable or doubtful cases, homeopaths avoid giving the high potencies and generally stick with the 30th or 200th, lest they stir things up too much. Alternatively, they may give a remedy that is related to the deep-acting *simillimum*, but which, because it is not the most similar, will not have as profound an effect on the patient's economy.

2. *Long aggravation with final and slow improvement.* Such a case is not quite as serious as the first. It may mean that the patient is beginning to undergo marked tissue change but has been caught just on the verge of being incurable. The eventual vital reaction after a long aggravation indicates that the patient still has sufficient vitality to be curable, although it is wise to proceed cautiously and not to administer the remedy in high potencies.

3. *Aggravation is quick, brief, and strong, followed by rapid improvement of the patient.* This reaction is highly desirable, indicating that the improvement will be long lasting and that no vital organs have undergone serious structural changes. With this kind of aggravation, there may be abscesses and suppurations of nonvital organs as the vital force throws off the illness through the more exterior, less vital organs. This is the sort of slight aggravation that is observed during the first hours after a remedy is given in an acute illness, or during the first few days in a chronic disease, and it is an excellent prognostic sign.

4. *No observable aggravation; steady recovery of the patient.* Such an outcome is ideal; it means that the remedy was correct and the potency selected was exactly suited to the case. The illness was not deep-seated and involved no organic changes. (This might also happen in a natural cure, without the aid of drugs.)

5. *First an amelioration, then an aggravation.* Either the remedy was only superficial and palliative, or the patient was incurable and the remedy only partially similar. In this case, it is necessary to reexamine the patient and to determine whether the aggravated symptoms can be traced to the remedy that was given. The symptoms may come back changed, and then a change of remedy will be called for. Sometimes, in the case of

an amelioration followed by an aggravation, homeopaths find that a deep-acting antimiasmatic remedy will be called for to enable the *simillimum* to take hold. This outcome after the administration of the remedy may also be the result of a placebo effect: the patient feels better immediately after the administration of the remedy, but once the reassurance obtained from seeing the doctor has worn off, the symptoms return worse than before.

6. *The amelioration of the symptoms is too short.* The patient must be questioned to see if he has done anything to-interfere with the action of the remedy, such as taking other drugs, using coffee or camphorated products that may antidote the remedy, or changing his living pattern in some way that interrupted the remedy's effect. In acute cases, the overly short amelioration may mean that the acute illness is progressing rapidly; the acute remedy may be "used up" quickly in such a condition, especially if it is a short-acting remedy. In a chronic case, amelioration should be relatively long lasting. When the amelioration is too brief, it may mean that organs have been destroyed or are threatened by the progress of the disease.

7. *Full-time amelioration of the symptoms without any special relief to the patient.* The patient cannot be fully cured, possibly owing to irreversible structural changes, and the case is open only to palliation.

8. *The symptoms turn out to be a proving of the remedy.* The patient may have an idiosyncrasy to the remedy given, or the patient may be oversensitive to all remedies. Such patients can present real difficulties in treatment, and Kent advises that they be treated with relatively lower potencies, the 30th and the 200th in acute cases, or the 30th, 200th, and 500th in chronic cases.

9. *The action of medicines on provers.* Kent observes that the constitutional state of a prover must be thoroughly evaluated before the proving so that the patient's constitutional symptoms can be subtracted from the symptoms exhibited in the proving. In healthy individuals, provings have a beneficial, tonic effect if they are properly conducted.

10. *New symptoms appear after the administration of the remedy.* The appearance of new symptoms, especially if there are a great number of them, generally indicates that the prescription was incorrect. Because the prescription was not homeopathic to the case, the new symptoms will eventually wear off, and the

patient will return to his original state, with no improvement or deterioration in his condition; however, if the new symptoms are exceedingly troublesome, the remedy may need to be antidoted.

11. *Old symptoms reappear.* There may first be an aggravation of the patient's symptoms, while the patient himself feels better. Whenever "new" symptoms appear after the administration of the remedy, the physician must inquire closely to determine whether these are actually old symptoms that preceded the patient's present state. When old symptoms begin to reappear in the reverse order of their coming (Hering's law), it is a sign that the patient is on the road to recovery. The physician must encourage the patient to make no attempt to treat these old symptoms as they come up, no matter how uncomfortable they may be. So long as the old symptoms come back and disappear, there should be no change in the medicine. The doctor must watch and wait, and if the old symptoms reappear and stay, the dose may need to be repeated.

12. *Symptoms take the wrong direction.* If the symptoms that appear after the administration of the remedy progress from external to internal, for example, instead of in the direction of Hering's law, it is a bad sign, and the more vital organs are threatened with structural change. In such a case the remedy must be antidoted immediately.

The Use of Placebo

The management of the patient can be an extremely difficult task for the homeopath. Especially in chronic diseases, the physician must be able to wait and observe, not giving a second prescription until he is sure that the effects of the first have exhausted themselves. The homeopath should educate his patient as to how homeopathic remedies work, so that the patient will not be tempted to undertake self-medication for annoying symptoms that may come up in the course of treatment. Particularly, the patient must be warned against the use of allopathic medications, nasal sprays, and rubs containing camphor or related substances. According to many homeopaths, the patient must also be advised not to drink coffee. Even the most well-educated patient, however, may have a hard time doing nothing while the remedy acts, and for this reason, homeopaths sometimes give "blank" tablets or powders of milk sugar (*saccharum lactis*) to their patients, to take at home as part of a regular schedule.[15] By giving the patient something to take, the homeopath is preventing him from interfering with the treatment by mixing the remedy with other drugs. Because it is administered while the patient is waiting out the action of a remedy, or while the homeopath is studying the case to make certain he will arrive at the *simillimum*, placebo is often called the "second-best remedy."

The Second Prescription

In our analysis of aggravations, we have already touched on some of the things that the homeopath may do after the first prescription has been given. By the first prescription, the homeopath means the first remedy that has acted. A homeopath may give a number of remedies, one after another, that have no effect, either because he has not taken the case correctly or because he has not made a thorough enough search for the *simillimum*; some cases have so few symptoms that it is difficult to settle on the correct remedy. At any rate, when we speak of the second prescription, we mean *the one that is given after one that has acted.*

There are, according to Kent, three possibilities for the second prescription: (1) a repetition of the first, (2) an antidote, or (3) a complementary remedy. It is always necessary for the physician to restudy a case before making the second prescription. The prime indication for a repetition of the first prescription is a return of the original symptoms. The physician must be very patient; he must be willing to merely watch and wait until he is certain that the first prescription has exhausted itself. Perhaps the patient has undergone steady improvement and now has come to a standstill; the physician must wait for a return of the original symptoms. If the original symptoms do reappear, it means

15. A similar situation exists with some allopathic birth control pills, where the last 5 days of a monthly "course" (28 pills) consist of nondrug compounds. This is done to remind women to take the pills on a daily basis.

that the first prescription was correct, that the case is curable, and that the second prescription must be a repetition of the first. It is common for homeopaths to repeat the first prescription in a different potency, generally a higher one, in order to reach the patient on a different dynamic plane. Sometimes the physician will run all the way up the range of potencies, finally returning to the original potency, before he can be certain that the original remedy will do no more for the patient.

If new symptoms appear, taking the place of the old symptoms, it is necessary to determine whether these new symptoms are actually old ones reappearing, in conformity with Hering's law. If these are genuinely new symptoms, the physician must look up the remedy to see if the symptoms resemble a proving of the remedy. If so, the prescription was not homeopathic to the case, and it must be antidoted if possible. In order to determine the antidotal second prescription, the doctor must take the case again and prescribe on the basis of the new symptoms, keeping the previous symptoms in mind but not giving them so much weight.

Sometimes the change of symptoms calls for a remedy that is complementary to the first prescription. There are many groupings of remedies that bear complementary relationships to each other, one remedy being acute and the other chronic. Sometimes after an acute remedy has been administered and has cleared up an acute illness, a new set of symptoms will emerge that will call for a different remedy— one that represents the chronic counterpart of the acute remedy. It is at the end of an acute illness that the constitutional state of the patient stands out most clearly, and often the chronic, or constitutional, remedy will be called for at this point, on the basis of the symptoms, to complete the case and prevent recurrences.

There is one further instance in which a change of remedy is called for, and that is when there is a mixture of two or more chronic miasms in the patient—where the first prescription has caused the symptoms of one miasm to pass off, and now the symptoms of a second, separate chronic miasm appear. In this case, there is a change in the plan of treatment, with the new prescription based on the symptoms that now predominate and that are connected with the previously submerged chronic miasm. This situation is related to the complex theory of chronic diseases.

THE THEORY OF CHRONIC DISEASES

With the publication of his *Chronic Diseases* in 1828, Hahnemann added another set of principles to the homeopathic doctrine. These new principles were based on more than a decade of observation, as well as extensive reading in the earlier medical literature. Hahnemann's theory of chronic diseases is an extremely difficult and, even today, controversial element of the homeopathic doctrine. Although not all contemporary homeopaths embrace completely Hahnemann's analysis, many find his observations useful in treating chronic cases.

Psora

What started Hahnemann on the road to his theory of chronic diseases was his observation that patients under treatment with a properly selected homeopathic remedy would show the expected improvement in their symptoms only to suffer a reappearance of their illness, perhaps in a changed form and with progressive worsening of their condition. Each new onslaught of disease would be removed homeopathically, yet the patient, under mental or physical stress, would continue to experience relapses and would gradually go downhill. Hahnemann began to suspect that such patients were suffering from a deeper-seated chronic disease that was being only partially manifested in each recurrence. He began to compile the symptomatology of the diseases that so recurred and to inquire closely of the patients about their medical histories, and he found in a vast number of such cases that the patient had somewhere early in his history an eruption of an itching skin condition, which had been suppressed either through medication or through some mechanical means. Searching the earlier literature, Hahnemann found evidence of chronic illnesses that had been preceded by suppressed cases of skin eruptions, and he concluded that the suppression had driven the miasm causing this itchy condition ever inward, and that, with each successive treatment of a new outcropping of the miasm, the disease was implanted deeper upon the economy. Hahnemann called this miasmatic disease *psora*, and he attributed most of the present illnesses of humanity to the suppression of the early manifestations of psora.

Hahnemann found evidence of psora in the epidemics of skin diseases of ancient times—plague, leprosy, and other serious afflictions—as well as in the apparently minor cases of "itch" in his own day. Because psora had developed over millennia, passed from one person to another not only through infection but also through heredity, and because in all its manifestations it had continually been subjected to suppression, Hahnemann believed that, in his time, it was so deeply implanted upon the economy of most of humankind that it could actually be considered the source of man's susceptibility to almost all diseases, acute and chronic.

Hahnemann claimed that at least seven-eighths of all the chronic maladies of man sprang from psora, and that the remaining one-eighth could be traced to the other two chronic miasms, the venereal miasms of syphilis and sycosis.

We should take a moment to look at the precise meaning of Hahnemann's term *psora*, since critics of homeopathy have taken great glee in ridiculing him for claiming that seven-eighths of humankind's ills could be traced to something called "the itch." First, note the similarity of this term to our current term *psoriasis*, which is recognized as one of the most intractable of skin diseases. Herbert A. Roberts, M.D., a homeopath writing in the 1940s, suggested that there may be a misunderstanding arising from the translation of Hahnemann's term. Whereas the Latin and Greek derivation of the word *psora* indicates that it means "scabies" or "psoriasis," Roberts suggests that Hahnemann derived his term from the Hebrew language, with which he was quite familiar, and that the true origin of the word is *tsorat* ("a groove," "a fault," "a pollution," "a stigma"). Thus, the word may have a more serious meaning than simply "the itch," although in many cases Hahnemann does point to the suppression of an itchy eruption as the beginning of the psoric pattern.

There is, furthermore, a hint of moralism in the discussion of psora by Hahnemann and his successors. They imply that psora is a symbolic manifestation of Original Sin, which established man's first susceptibility to disease:

Hence this state, the state of the human mind and the state of the human body, is a state of susceptibility to disease from willing evils, from thinking that which is false and making life one continuous heredity of false things, and so this form of disease, psora, is but an outward manifestation of that which is prior in man. . . .

The human race today walking the face of the earth is but little better than a moral leper. Such is the state of the human mind at the present day. To put it another way, everyone is psoric.[16]

Be that as it may, Hahnemann, having compiled voluminous symptoms associated with latent psora and its outbreaks in the form of various chronic diseases, began his search for remedies whose symptom pictures most closely fit the complex symptom image of psora. Primary among the antipsoric remedies was sulfur, which has in its pathogenesis many skin eruptions, as well as other symptoms. Although Hahnemann considered sulfur the preeminent antipsoric remedy, he also classed a large number of other remedies as antipsoric, and he proceeded to establish their antipsoric qualities by administering them, on the basis of similarity, to patients with chronic diseases. When the patient's symptoms were removed, to be replaced with earlier, more primitive manifestations of psora, which were then likewise removed, he felt he had confirmation of the antipsoric action of such remedies.

Although the chronic miasm of psora has innumerable symptoms, it is characteristic of the psoric state that psora alone does not produce destruction of tissue, expressing itself more in surface symptoms and functional and mental symptoms.

16. Kent, *Lectures on Homeopathic Philosophy*, p. 147.

The Venereal Miasms: Syphilis and Sycosis

The case is quite different with the two other chronic miasms, which Hahnemann identified as *syphilis* and *sycosis*. Syphilis, as we know, has its first manifestation in a characteristic chancre at the site of contagion, and if untreated progresses through secondary and tertiary stages, eventually resulting in the destruction of nervous and connective tissue, including the bones and cartilage. Sycosis is the chronic miasmatic form of gonorrhea and is to be distinguished from the acute form of gonorrhea which, if treated, will not implant itself upon the economy in the form of the sycotic miasm. The sycotic stigma is initially a "fig wart," a whitish wartlike skin growth, but when this growth is suppressed through medicines or excision, the homeopath believes that the miasm is driven inward, finally expressing itself in a characteristic overgrowth of tissue (warts, excessive hair, etc.).

Like psora, sycosis and syphilis are contagious and capable of being passed on through heredity. According to homeopaths, a peculiar quality of the venereal miasms is that when they are transmitted from one person to another through infection, they are transmitted in the stage of development at which they are present in the transmitter. Thus, a woman infected by a man whose sycotic miasm had reached a secondary stage would receive the sycosis in the secondary stage; she would never have the characteristic fig wart, and in the course of cure it would not be necessary for a fig wart to appear and subsequently disappear for her cure to be complete.

Furthermore, the three chronic miasms can be combined, resulting in cases that are especially difficult to cure. Psora may be combined with either sycosis or syphilis, or all three may be mixed up in one case, producing the gravest sorts of illnesses. In curing such a case, it is necessary to administer an antipsoric, on the basis of manifest symptoms, until the psoric symptoms pass off and the symptoms of the underlying sycotic or syphilitic miasm emerge; these are then treated with the appropriate antimiasmatic drug on the basis of the new symptoms, and so forth, zigzagging the patient to a cure.

Hahnemann determined the antisycotic and antisyphilitic remedies in the same way that he did the antipsorics, by compiling the symptomatology of each miasm, studying the pathogenesis of remedies to find the ones that were similar to the composite pictures, and then administering the remedies to patients suffering from each of the miasms and watching the progress of symptoms. Although Hahnemann classed a number of remedies as antisycotic or antisyphilitic, he felt that mercury was the principal antisyphilitic remedy and *Thuja* (arborvitae) the antisycotic of primary importance.

Current Application of the Theory of Chronic Diseases

In identifying specific remedies for the three chronic miasms, Hahnemann seems to have deviated from his earlier tenet of individualizing each case and to have moved in the direction of the "disease entity." Despite this apparent doctrinal deviation, there is general agreement among homeopaths that Hahnemann's description of the three chronic miasms, with their characteristic manifestations and their ways of combining with one another, is correct. There is less agreement as to whether there is an actual causal relationship between the acute forms of the diseases and the chronic miasms for which they are named. In practice, many homeopaths stick to prescribing on the basis of obvious similarity, without searching for evidence of an underlying chronic miasm. Many, however, will apply Hahnemann's theory of chronic diseases when they find a case failing to respond to a carefully selected remedy; in such a case they will search for an antimiasmatic remedy that matches the patient's symptoms, and they often find that, after the administration of the antimiasmatic, the indicated remedy for an acute disease will be effective once again. For example, many cases that have come to a standstill, in which the patient is not responding to the indicated remedy, will respond to the proper remedies once again after a dose of sulfur has been given.

Constitutional Prescribing

From the foregoing discussion it can be seen that homeopaths may prescribe for chronic conditions without strict adherence to Hahnemann's theory of chronic diseases, and many of them will have recourse to this theory only when it seems to be the best way to unravel a case. Patients can be treated with constitutional remedies—that is, chronic remedies chosen on the basis of their similarity to the clear constitutional symptomatology of the patient—without attaching a specific miasmatic name to the patient's constitutional condition. It happens that many of the most frequently employed constitutional remedies are antimiasmatics, but the prescriber need not go deeply into the theory of chronic diseases in order to determine the constitutional remedy. Because constitutional treatment builds up the patient's resistance to attacks of acute disease, as well as clearing up chronic conditions, constitutional prescribing is a preventative as well as a curative approach in homeopathy.

3

HOMEOPATHY IN FIRST AID AND MINOR ILLNESSES

GUIDELINES TO PRACTICAL APPLICATIONS

Since the most convincing evidence for the correctness of the homeopathic approach must be its results in actual use, this chapter will describe some common applications in easily recognized emergency situations and in some minor ailments. The best way to evaluate homeopathic practice is under the guidance of a homeopathic practitioner, and even the simple remedies described below should only be administered after experienced consultation. We cannot guarantee, of course, that the remedies mentioned will be effective, and it must always be borne in mind that the homeopathic remedies are given in addition to usual first aid procedures, which must never be neglected. To fully understand homeopathy, however, some practical experience *is* necessary, and if you decide to try some of these remedies, you will need a supply of them. Chapter 6 contains a detailed list of the more common remedies, and Appendix C lists some homeopathic pharmacies and mail-order suppliers. Homeopathic first aid kits are available through a number of suppliers, or you may want to assemble your own kit on the basis of the information provided in this chapter.

You will notice that there is not always a complete symptom image of the patient for each of the kinds of injuries or illnesses described below. This may appear to be a departure from the homeopathic principle of looking at the patient as a whole. However, in first aid situations particularly, and to a lesser extent in the minor ailments we shall describe, the symptomatic condition of the patient is dependent to a large degree on the nature of the emergency or acute ailment. In the treatment of most acute illnesses, or in constitutional prescribing, a much more complete symptom picture of the patient must be obtained before a homeopathic remedy can be selected. This is why such applications of homeopathy are restricted to practitioners who have extensive training and clinical experience. On the other hand, in first aid situations, by the very nature of the emergency, there is generally no doctor present, and the use of homeopathic remedies in addition to normal first aid procedures may help stabilize the patient's condition until professional attention can be obtained. The homeopathic remedies may also speed recovery.

The following material is drawn from the writings and clinical experience of contemporary homeopathic practitioners. Recommended dosages vary somewhat among practitioners. Generally the 30th is suggested in this chapter; this medium potency is preferred among prescribers who regularly use the high potencies in many conditions. Also, the 30th is the highest potency available over the counter to laypeople. Because the 30th represents a level of dilution beyond the limit of Avogadro's number, it can also provide evidence of the activity of the ultramolecular dose.

Frequency of dosage is also indicated. This represents the consensus as to how often a given remedy should be repeated in a certain situation. It is important to remember that information about repetition of doses represents the *most often* a remedy should be given. *As long as the patient feels relief, the remedy is not repeated.* This rule is of paramount importance in the application of homeopathy.

The number of tablets or pillules you take in a single dose is relatively unimportant. It is the potency, the energetic pattern, of the remedy that is important. According to most practitioners, two or three tablets should be sufficient. Some homeopaths even report astonishing results when the patient simply *sniffs* the remedy from an unstoppered bottle, but, given our society's predilection for taking something, you might feel a little less skeptical if you actually allow a couple of tablets to dissolve on or under your tongue. Since they are made of sugar, they dissolve readily; they do not need to be washed down with water. In normal homeopathic practice, patients are advised not to eat or drink anything half an hour to an hour before and after taking the remedy. In emergencies, however, such precautions are not always possible.

Homeopaths also advise against the use of certain substances when taking a homeopathic remedy. Especially prohibited are any preparations containing camphor, since camphor is believed to interfere with the action of remedies. Chest rubs and similar camphorated products should therefore be avoided when remedies are given. Similarly, homeopaths recommend that no allopathic drugs be given when the patient is receiving a homeopathic remedy. Coffee is also believed to antidote remedies, and some practitioners advise their patients not to drink any coffee at all if they are under constitutional homeopathic treatment. If you are a heavy coffee drinker and decide not to drink it while taking a homeopathic remedy, you might experience such benefits from not drinking coffee that your results will be somewhat difficult to interpret!

In some situations, as in mechanical injuries, the indications for a remedy are purely physical. This does not mean that the remedy itself has no mental symptoms in its provings, but simply that in the case described the remedy can be determined on physical indications alone. In other situations the mental component is of primary importance, or serves to distinguish between conditions calling for different remedies. This will give you some idea of how mental and physical symptoms are linked in the theory and practice of homeopathy.

Hopefully, you will not be involved often in the first aid situations described below. In order to provide another kind of opportunity for evaluating homeopathy, we have described some minor ailments that you might ordinarily treat with over-the-counter allopathic medications. The next time you suffer from such a minor ailment, you may want to try the homeopathic remedies indicated. Remember, however, that homeopathic prescribing becomes much more complex when we get into the area of acute diseases, no matter how minor. For example, there are a number of remedies used by homeopaths for the common cold, depending on the reaction of the patient to taking cold, the exciting cause of the cold, etc. Patients can also be treated constitutionally for colds, or receive no specific acute treatment while under the influence of a constitutional remedy. Unless your particular ailment corresponds extremely closely to the symptoms described, the indicated remedy will probably not be much help. If a remedy is well indicated, however, you may gain convincing evidence of the relief that homeopathic remedies can provide, and you will also have freed yourself from dependence on the suppressive allopathic drugs you may have been using in the past.

HOMEOPATHY IN FIRST AID

Shock

To a greater or lesser degree, shock occurs with any accident or sudden illness. It results from a disturbance in the blood circulation, owing to blood loss or other causes. Because of the reduced volume of blood returning to the heart, the nervous system and other tissues do not receive an adequate supply of the oxygen carried by the blood. The patient becomes pale, with cold, clammy skin. The pulse is rapid and becomes progressively weaker. Breathing is shallow. The patient is restless and apprehensive.

Shock is a serious condition, and conventional first aid measures should be taken immediately. The patient should be reassured and his fear allayed, since fear will aggravate the condition. He should be kept lying flat, with clothing loosened. Warm coverings should be used, for cold will make the patient worse, but avoid overheating. Allow the patient to get plenty of fresh air.

We have chosen to treat the problem of shock first as a way of introducing two of the great homeopathic first aid remedies: *Arnica* and Aconite. One of these remedies is often recommended as the first to be given after accidents, followed by remedies suited to the specific injury. For treating shock by itself, the remedies can be distinguished by the following indications:

Arnica is given for shock from any injury involving bleeding, physical blows, falls, etc. It relieves pain, bleeding, and shock symptoms. The patient may be confused and mentally dull, almost comatose, and he may rouse himself to push the doctor away, saying he doesn't need a doctor when he obviously does. Even if the patient is unconscious, *Arnica* can be placed on the tongue. *Arnica* 30 is given every hour until better.

Aconite is given for shock with fear. The patient is anxious, fearful, restless after the injury. He may be so certain he is going to die that he will predict the time of his death. Aconite is an excellent remedy for patients who have suffered severe burns, auto collisions, or other frightening trauma, as the allaying of their fears will help to counteract the effects of shock. Aconite 30 is given every hour until the patient is better.

Bruises

The familiar signs of pain, swelling, and many hued skin discoloration results from damage to the soft tissues beneath the skin, with resultant extravasation of blood. Be alert for signs of internal bleeding or organ damage, particularly with blows to the head, chest, or abdomen. Cold or ice compresses will reduce the swelling.

Arnica 200 is recommended as an immediate dose. If 200 is not available, give *Arnica* 30 two or three times a day for a few days, according to the severity of the bruising. *Arnica* is said to relieve pain and promote reabsorption of blood.

Ledum 12 or 6 may be given after *Arnica* if there is a delay in the disappearance of the bruise, especially if the affected part feels cold and numb and is relieved by cold applications. *Ledum* is considered the best remedy for black eyes, providing immediate relief of pain and reducing subsequent discoloration.

Ruta is given for bone bruises or injuries of the periosteum (the tissue covering bone).

Arnica lotion, made of five drops of *Arnica* tincture to one-half pint of cold water, may be applied in external compresses to bruises and to muscles that are bruised or tired from overexertion. *Do not apply Arnica to skin that is* scratched or cut, as it can produce *Arnica* poisoning. *Do not leave compresses on too long*, for some people are very sensitive to this remedy.

Cuts

If the skin has been cut by a sharp instrument or torn raggedly, underlying structures, including blood vessels, nerves, muscles, or tendons, may have been injured. Bleeding can be controlled by local pressure or with a tourniquet when there is arterial spurting that cannot be controlled by pressure. Great caution must be used with a tourniquet; make sure you loosen it at half-hour intervals. For deep cuts, immediate surgical assistance will be required to rejoin the damage structures and close the skin edges.

For *minor clean cuts*, allow a little bleeding to cleanse the wound from within.

Calendula or *Hypericum* lotion (ten drops of the tincture to a half-pint of cold water) is used externally to moisten the dressing, and a bandage is applied to bring the wound edges together. These two remedies promote the healing of the wound and combat infection, so allopathic antiseptic preparations need not be used. The dressing may be moistened by dropping fresh lotion on the outside of the dressing on the first day.

Staphisagria 30 is a commonly used homeopathic remedy for cuts caused by sharp instruments that produce stinging, smarting pain.

Calendula 30 may be given internally twice a day, in combination with the external dressing, to help the healing process.

For *severe lacerated wounds* that are ragged, or where there has been extensive damage to underlying tissues, surgical attention may be required, but the following may be given in the interim:

Arnica 200, one or two doses. Or *Arnica* 30.

Hypericum lotion (ten drops to a half-pint of cold water) may be applied externally.

With severe wounds, there is frequently injury to nerves, so the recommended remedy after *Arnica* is *Hypericum* three times a day; or, if the pain is severe, *Hypericum* 30 every hour or so until the patient feels relief. The characteristic pain calling for *Hypericum* is shooting pain going centrally through the affected limb.

Arnica 6 may be given twice a day thereafter, the number of days depending on the severity of the injury. *Arnica* is said to help speed up the healing.

Puncture Wounds

In puncture wounds caused by sharp objects, the skin may not be badly damaged, but underlying structures may be injured and infection may be implanted deep in the tissue. The possibility of tetanus must be considered in puncture wounds, and if the patient has not had a recent tetanus toxoid inoculation, it should be administered by a physician. Puncture wounds to the abdomen or chest are particularly apt to involve organ damage and hemorrhage, and medical attention should be obtained.

Ledum 30 is the preferred homeopathic remedy for puncture wounds, and it is reputed to prevent tetanus; without the advice of a homeopathic physician, however, do not neglect to obtain a tetanus toxoid shot. *Ledum* also promotes the healing of wounds in parts of the body that are rich in nerves. It is given three times a day for two or three days. The *Ledum* patient is chilly, and the wounded parts feel cold to touch; the pains are better with cold applications and worse with warm applications.

Hypericum is another remedy for puncture wounds. It also helps in injuries to nerves. *Hypericum* 6 may be given after the above course of *Ledum; Hypericum* is especially indicated if the wound is painful, or if there are pains shooting up the injured limb. However, if the injured part remains cold and numb or is sensitive to touch and better with cold, *Ledum* should be continued in 6 rather than changing to *Hypericum*.

Crushing Injuries

Hypericum 30 is recommended for injuries to nerves or to parts of the body that are richly supplied with nerves, so it is useful in treating crushed fingertips or toes, particularly if the injured area is sensitive to touch.

Surgical and Dental Operations

Of course, operations are not accidental, but because they involve bleeding and injury to tissues, homeopathic remedies can be of help.

Arnica is the primary remedy for operations, given in the 30th before and after surgery to promote healing. *Arnica* is also given in the higher potencies—for wounds that have not healed well or for patients who have not felt well since an operation.

Aconite 30 may be given before an operation if the patient shows apprehension; it is especially useful for children or fearful adults. It can also be helpful after an operation if the patient is restless and tosses about in bed.

Hypericum 200 can also be given the morning before an operation; *Hypericum*'s special affinity is for parts richly supplied with nerves.

Staphisagria may be useful after surgical operations for wounds that are painful, stinging, and smarting.

For dental operations, homeopathic remedies can also help to reduce pain and may allow the patient to have his teeth drilled with no Novocain, or a reduced dose. Because many of the allopathic anesthetics used in dental procedures can antidote homeopathic remedies, the following remedies are of special importance for patients who are under constitutional homeopathic treatment:

Hypericum 200, given just before drilling, may allow the patient to reduce his dose of Novocain, or he may not need it at all.

Calendula lotion (ten drops to a half-pint of cold water) is useful as a mouthwash after tooth extraction, since it reduces the risk of infection, promotes the proper healing of wounds, and helps control bleeding.

Childbirth

Most remedies used to prepare women for childbirth are constitutional and not within the scope of this chapter. However, *Arnica*, given right before delivery, makes the birth quicker and less painful and speeds the mother's recovery after delivery. *Arnica* is also recommended for the newborn infant, for it promotes recovery from the trauma of birth and may reduce the risk of damage to the infant in difficult deliveries.

Sprains and Strains

Sprains and strains, caused by sudden twists and turns, are injuries to muscles and to the ligaments that attach muscle to bone. Pain, disability, and local swelling owing to effusion of fluid quickly follow such injuries. It is wise to have a physician check for fracture in severe injuries of this type.

Arnica is given internally as soon as possible after a sprain or strain, the 30th every hour for five or six doses. *Arnica* lotion (five drops tincture to a half-pint cold water) may be applied as a moist compress with a firm bandage to support the injured limb. Be careful, however, not to apply *Arnica* lotion if the skin is broken. For damage to muscle, with bruising, *Arnica* 6 is considered the best remedy. Athletes rub down with *Arnica* lotion before and after practice to prevent stiffness and soreness from overexertion.

Rhus toxicodendron (*Rhus tox.*) is given after *Arnica*, in the 12th or 6th, two or three times a day until the injury is better. *Rhus tox.* is also valued as a preventative in activities that produce stiffness, such as gardening. It can be taken before working and then afterwards and is reputed to prevent pain and stiffness.

Ruta is recommended for sprains and dislocations, synovitis, and inflammation of ligaments, knee joints, and wrist joints. If the injury is close to the bone, and the periosteum (bone covering) is damaged, *Ruta* is the remedy of choice; the 6 is preferred. *Ruta* is a deeper-acting remedy than *Rhus tox.* and is used where the injury is more severe— where tendons have been wrenched, ligaments split, or periosteum or bone bruised. *Ruta* is given for tennis elbow.

Both *Rhus tox.* 6 and *Ruta* 6 are used for chronic sprains that result from repeated motions that are mildly injurious, such as certain occupational activities that have a cumulative effect of producing local pain over a muscle attachment and pain on certain movements. Of course, the cause of the repeated irritation should be identified and the activity avoided.

For pains in the heel tendons, *Ruta* is better than *Rhus tox.*

Ledum is used for sprains in people who have weak ankles and feet, who are always spraining their ankles. If the affected part is cold and numb, better with cold applications and worse with heat, *Ledum* 6 is the preferred remedy.

Bryonia 30, three times a day, is given for sprains and strains if the joint near the injury is swollen and distended with fluid or painful with the slightest movement. Once the swelling has gone down, *Bryonia* is followed with *Rhus tox.* 6.

Fractures

Usually, but not always, there will be obvious deformity when a bone is broken. Whenever fracture is suspected, extreme care must be taken not to move the broken fragments; a splint may be used. Almost all fractures will have pain, swelling, tenderness over the bone, and some disability.

Arnica 200, one or two doses, is given immediately after the injury, followed by *Arnica* 30 or *Ledum* 30 two or three times a day for a few days to help absorb the extravasated blood and reduce swelling.

Symphytum 6 follows the above remedies and is given for any fracture to speed the union of broken bones. Given once a day for a week or two, *Symphytum* is used especially for fractures of the long bones. There may be a peculiar prickling pain, or pain along the shaft or periosteum of the broken bone which is often noticed following fracture. Persistent nonunion and accompanying disability are also treated with *Symphytum.*

Calc. Phos. 30, twice a week, is given for fractures in elderly people. Valuable in nonunion of bones, it is continued for several weeks.

Ruta may be given if the fractured bone is greatly injured or bruised and there is an aching, bruised feeling of the whole body. It is also useful for fractured ribs, given in three doses, one every other day.

Burns

Minor burns will result only in redness of the skin. More severe burn will produce blistering or actual charring of the skin. Serum loss occurs through the pouring of fluids through the burned surface, increasing shock and depriving the body of vital substances. There is danger of infection. The patient should be treated for shock if present. A dressing should be placed over the exposed burned area without disturbing any burned clothing, and the patient should be kept warmly covered in a well-ventilated room. Sweating will increase fluid loss, so overheating should be avoided.

Homeopaths tell us that the best immediate first aid measure for minor burns is to expose the burned part to heat until the pain becomes bearable. This procedure is considered far preferable to putting the burned part in cold water, since once the cold water is removed the pain is only intensified.

For minor first-degree burns, a dressing moistened with *Urtica urens* lotion (tincture in water) is recommended, especially for any pain with burns. *Urtica* is also available as an ointment. *Hypericum* lotion or *Calendula* lotion (ten drops of tincture to a half-pint of cold water) may also be used, particularly for their antiseptic properties.

Urtica urens 30 is also given internally for minor burns. For second-degree burns, where there is blistering present, *Causticum* 30 may be given internally, the *Hypericum* as a lotion externally. After the initial healing, *Calendula* lotion is given to prevent scarring.

For severe burns, particularly third-degree burns where the skin is charred, *Arnica* is given first for shock (200 is the recommended dose), or aconite if the patient is suffering from fright. *Cantharis* 30 may then be given every ten minutes or so until the patient feels relief from the pain. *Urtica* 30 is another remedy given for relief of pain from severe burns.

Heatstroke

Heatstroke, or sunstroke, is a profound failure of the body's heat-regulating mechanism owing to exposure to high temperatures. The patient's temperature rises to dangerously high levels; the skin is hot and dry, the pulse rate increased. The warning symptoms of heatstroke are lassitude, headache, giddiness, nausea, and diminution of sweating. Circulatory collapse, cramps or convulsions, and coma may follow. Immediate measures should be taken—cold sponging and fanning—to reduce the patient's temperature to 101° F. The patient should be kept in a cool place, off the ground, with her head kept high and constantly cooled.

Glonoin, or nitroglycerin, is the preferred homeopathic remedy for sunstroke or heatstroke, and it is also used as a preventive. If glonoin is given on a regular basis at the start of the summer, it is believed to build up resistance to heat. It is given this way by homeopaths to prepare children for prolonged exposure to the sun at summer camps.

For someone who actually has a case of heatstroke, a potentially fatal condition, the preferred remedy is glonoin 6, 12, or 30, a few doses each hour or half hour until improvement is obvious.

Sunburn

Glonoin 200, one per hour for three doses, is given for sunburn. *Calendula* lotion may be applied externally.

Food Poisoning

Arsenicum album is a highly valued first aid remedy for the severe diarrhea that appears after eating food that has been contaminated with *Salmonella*; the patient is pale, vomiting, thirsty, prostrated, and anxious. Both *Arsenicum* and nux vomica are common remedies for travelers with "turista."

Head Injuries

Arnica 30 every half hour for five or six doses is given immediately after a head injury. *Arnica* is also used in old head injuries that still bother the patient.

Natrum sulphuricum 30 is another remedy for persistent effects of head injuries, such as recurrent headaches. In the 200 potency it is also used for posttraumatic syndromes, in which there is a history of head injury or concussion in the past. This remedy has also been used to overcome the ill effects of forceps deliveries in which the head of the infant was traumatized.

Spinal Injuries

Hypericum is the recommended homeopathic remedy for mechanical injuries to the spinal cord that have been caused by falls, etc. The 30th is given two or three times daily for a few days. *Arnica* 200, one or two doses, may be given first to prevent persistent symptoms. *Arnica* is also used to alleviate the effects of old spinal injuries.

Insect Bites

There are innumerable species of insects to which some people may have adverse reactions. Hypersensitive people can be killed by the bite of a single relatively harmless insect. Among the more common homeopathic remedies for insect bites are the following:

Ledum is useful for animal poisons in general, and for insect stings and bites, especially mosquitoes and bee venom. *Ledum* helps to reduce swelling, alleviate pain, and counteract the effects of the poison. For a severe local reaction, *Ledum* 200 is used, one or two doses; if less severe, *Ledum* 30 is used for a few doses, or *Ledum* 6 for more prolonged use. *Ledum* bites are cold, numb, sensitive to touch, and relieved with cold applications.

For people who are allergic to spider bites, when there is a radiating red reaction around the area of the bite, *Ledum* or *Rhus Tox.* is recommended.

Apis 30 is given for burning, stinging bites where there is rapid swelling, as is characteristic of the bite of the honeybee from which it is derived. *Urtica urens* is also used for beestings.

Hypericum 30 to 6 is given for bites when there is pain shooting up the limb. If the part is red and angry looking, with burning pain, *Cantharis* 30 may be given.

Carbolicum acidum 30 is used for severe allergic reactions to beestings; if the symptoms are very serious, it is given every half hour.

It is said that *Staphisagria* 12, given ahead of time, will help keep mosquitoes away.

For treatment of wasp sting, *Arnica* tincture, applied to the bite, is said to cure the sting at once. *Ledum* tincture is also used.

For beesting, use tincture of *Ledum*, *Urtica urens*, or *Apis*, applied externally.

For gnat bites, use *Calendula* tincture or *Hypericum* tincture, applied externally.

Stroke and Heart Attack

Because we may have occasion to help someone afflicted with one of these all too prevalent problems, it is good to be able to recognize the signs of stroke and heart attack and to know what remedies homeopaths recommend to be given immediately, before help arrives. Heart attack is relatively simple to recognize because the patient will show evidence of severe chest pain, with or without radiation into the arm or other parts of the body.

Stroke may be more subtle. A stroke, or cerebrovascular accident, comes about either because a blood vessel bursts in the skull or because a clot blocks a blood vessel. The blood supply is cut off to a portion of the brain, resulting in symptoms ranging from mild to severe. The patient may simply experience a sudden weakness in a limb, numbness, or confusion of speech or thought. The patient should immediately be put in bed and reassured, and a doctor should be called. In severe cases, the patient may lose consciousness. He should not be moved, but should be kept covered, and if he is comatose, his head should be turned to one side to prevent inhalation of vomit or blood into his windpipe.

Arnica is highly praised as an immediate remedy for heart attack. Homeopaths believe that many more lives could be saved if medics carried *Arnica* in ambulances.

For stroke, Aconite 30 in a few doses is helpful to allay anxiety, followed by *Arnica* 30 two or three times a day for a few days to help the healing of the brain injury and the reabsorption of the blood clot. In more severe cases, when the patient is unconscious, a dose of *Arnica* 200 may be placed under the tongue.

Opium 30 is another remedy used for comatose patients whose faces are dusky and flushed and who breathe noisily, puffing out their cheeks on each expiration.

REMEDIES FOR SOME COMMON AILMENTS
The Common Cold

Because just about everyone catches cold at some time or other, you may want to see how homeopathic remedies can help in this common ailment. It is important to remember that cold symptoms may be the result of the body's adjustment to changes in climate or weather conditions. It is advisable not to suppress every little sniffle with medicines of any kind, but rather to let such minor illnesses run their course, thereby conferring upon the body a greater degree of resistance to climatic change. Such allopathic drugs as antihistamines may actually change the condition of the mucous membranes and cause the symptoms to hang on longer, in suppressed or altered form.

During the course of a cold, the symptoms may change, and in that case a change of remedy will be called for. Where they are clearly indicated, the following homeopathic remedies may be given in the 30th every four hours for a day or two. Some remedies, such as Aconite, are recommended only for the very.earliest stages of a cold.

Traditionally, the remedy of choice at the very first signs of a cold has been Aconite, especially when the cold is of sudden onset after exposure to cold dry wind, and in patients who are of robust constitutions. The cold starts just a few hours after exposure. There is much sneezing and running of the nose; the discharge is clear and hot. The throat may be red and inflamed, and the mucous membranes generally dry, burning, and smarting. There may be a roaring in the ears. The patient may be thirsty. The Aconite cold is marked by a rapid rise in temperature, and the patient may be anxious and restless. Symptoms are worse in a stuffy room and at night. Because Aconite is of brief action, it is generally recommended only during the first twenty-four hours after this rapid pattern of onset, and it is to be given on the first sneeze or shiver, especially after exposure to dry cold. If taken frequently in the first stages of a cold when properly indicated, Aconite is reputed to clear up cold symptoms in twenty-four hours.

At the present time, homeopaths are not always experiencing the same success with Aconite that was reported by earlier prescribers. Perhaps the change in the population's susceptibility to this remedy can be attributed to the influence of changes in our diet and contaminants in our environment—as well as the results of widespread allopathic drugging—that were not present in earlier times.

A present-day remedy that is held to be very useful in the first stages of a cold is *Ferrum phosphoricum. Ferrum phos.* 30 may be given in the early stages of a cold that does not have marked indications. The patient is simply not feeling well, without any real symptoms. *Ferrum phos.* can be called a "precold" remedy, and it is particularly likely to be helpful after exposure to dampness. In children with a tendency to croup, the croup is said to develop less frequently if *Ferrum phos.* is given at the first signs of not feeling well. In more advanced cases, *Ferrum phos.* is associated with colds that go into the chest quickly, with pleural involvement, stabbing pain in the chest, and sore muscles in the chest wall, worse with motion. The patient wants to lie quietly and is sensitive to noise. He is thirsty for large quantities of cold liquids. The tongue is uncoated and may be dark, red, and inflamed. There is an irritating, persistent cough associated with soreness in the chest. Symptoms are generally worse from motion, better from cold.

As a cold progresses beyond the premonitory symptoms, a second group of remedies is called for. In this stage, two remedies are widely recommended: *Arsenicum album* if the patient is cold, and *Belladonna* if the patient is hot.

In the *Arsenicum* stage, the cold has set in and the patient is sneezing and feels chilly. He wants warmth, but his head feels better in open air. There is a watery, burning discharge from the nose that excoriates the upper lip, and the nose may be stuffed up all the time. The patient sneezes frequently because of an irritable spot in the nose. There is a dry, wheezing, hacking cough, with no expectoration. The patient has burning pains, better from heat. The *Arsenicum* type of cold tends to spread quickly to the chest, and if *Arsenicum* is given it may prevent chest involvement.

The *Belladonna* patient is very hot. *Belladonna* is recommended for colds that come on with violent onset after exposure to chilling. The cold begins with a raw, red throat; the nose is swollen, red, and sore. There is little discharge; the mucous membranes are dry. The patient is flushed and very thirsty. There may be a violent, pulsating headache and a dry, tearing cough that scrapes the throat and causes hoarseness. The patient is flushed and hot. Hoarseness; larynx painful and dry. The inflammation has a tendency to be right-sided, or that may start on the right and spread to the left. There is rapid progress of symptoms. A characteristic feature of *Belladonna* is the crestlike pattern of pains and aggravations: symptoms appear suddenly, build in intensity, then disappear suddenly. This pattern of aggravation may be enough to indicate *Belladonna* even if the patient is not red, hot, and dry.

As a cold becomes more developed, another group of remedies is called for, including the following:

Hepar sulphuris calcareum is given for a cold that comes on after exposure to cold, dry weather. There is a characteristic sticking sensation, like a splinter, at the back of the throat, and in the early stages there may be a paroxysmal, dry, teasing cough. There is much sneezing, especially in cold wind. The discharge is watery at first but later becomes thick, yellow, and offensive. The patient is chilly, but he sweats a lot without relief, and he is irritable and hypersensitive to touch, pain, and drafts. The *hepar* cold affects the nose, ears, throat, and chest, and the patient may have a croupy cough. If *hepar* is given early, it can prevent the development of bronchitis.

For persistent colds that have settled in the nose, *Pulsatilla* is one of the mainstays of homeopathy. In this type of cold the nasal discharge is thick, yellow, and bland. The nose is stopped up at night and in the house, and the flow becomes copious in the morning and out of doors. There is a loss of the senses of smell and taste, and there may be chills up and down the back.

For persistent colds affecting the throat, phosphorus is a useful remedy. The phosphorus cold begins in the throat or chest. Sneezing causes pain in the throat or head. The nose is alternately running and blocked, or one nostril may be stopped up and the other running. The nose is sore, red, and shiny. There is hoarseness and sore throat and a feeling of tightness in the chest with a tight, racking cough that is worse on going from a warm room into open air.

Other cold remedies, described below, may be called for in the later stages of a cold, as the symptoms change and point to them. Some remedies can be identified according to the conditions under which the cold was contracted, or the first symptoms manifested in the cold.

The remedy *Allium cepa*, or the common onion, is recommended for colds whose symptoms are familiar to anyone who has cut up this vegetable. The patient's eyes are red and watering with a bland discharge. The nose has a profuse, acrid discharge which burns the nose and upper lip; the throat and chest may also become raw. There is paroxysmal sneezing and a cough that seems to tear the larynx. There may be a sensation of thickness in the head, and the patient is hot, thirsty, and headachy.

Bryonia alba is useful in colds whose onset is delayed, with slowly developing symptoms that finally settle in the chest. *Bryonia* is given for colds that begin with sneezing, watery nasal discharge, and red, watery eyes. The cold goes to the throat and larynx, causing hoarseness, and then moves into the lungs, with bronchitis. There is a painful, dry, spasmodic cough that shakes the whole body. Severe headache. The patient may hold his chest or head when he coughs because of the pain accompanying coughing. He is hot and thirsty for large quantities of cold drinks. The mucous membranes are dry. The patient wants to be left alone, lying perfectly still. He may have a heavy,. bluish appearance. *Bryonia* is good for colds with long-standing coughs, and often follows *Gelsemium* (see below).

Causticum is used in colds that start with dryness and rawness in the back of the throat and develop into hoarseness and loss of voice. There is a dry, tickling cough with little expectoration. Mucous collects in the back of the throat; the patient tries to dislodge it but often has to swallow it. There is morning sneezing and stuffiness of the nose. Often there is frequency of urination with these colds, and there may be urinary incontinence upon sneezing, coughing, or blowing the nose. The eyes water on going into the open air, with much blinking. The upper eyelids may be heavy.

The *Gelsemium* cold is delayed in onset, coming on days after exposure in warm, moist weather, or after changes in the weather. The patient may have a history of feeling chilled after being overheated some days previously. *Gelsemium* is a remedy for the "summer cold," and for influenza-type colds or colds during mild winters. Although the patient has chills and shivers up and down the spine, he feels hot and sticky; or he may feel hot and cold alternately. He feels better sitting by a source of heat. The fluid discharge from the nose makes the nostrils sore. There is headache and a feeling of aching and heaviness all over, especially in the eyelids and limbs. There may be a tickling, tearing cough, or a more croupy kind of cough. The patient does not want to be disturbed. There is a heavy, bluish appearance similar to the early stages of *Bryonia*, and *Bryonia* often follows *Gelsemium*.

Mercurius is used for colds that begin with creeping chilliness. There is violent sneezing. The discharge from the nose is fluent, corrosive, greenish, and offensive. The nose is red, shiny, and sore. The sinuses may have catarrhal inflammation. The throat may be sore, with hoarseness of voice. Tickling cough, worse from both heat and cold. Metallic, sweet, or salty taste in mouth. Profuse offensive sweats that do not relieve symptoms. Tongue is flabby, swollen, bearing imprint of teeth.

Nux vomica is given for colds that come on after exposure to dry, cold weather. There is much sneezing, associated with an irritating raw spot high in the back of the nostril. The nose may be blocked or running, stuffed up at night and running in a warm room or during the day; better out of doors. A painful, teasing, spasmodic cough may develop. There may be pain in the larynx and a tearing feeling in the chest on coughing. In this type of cold, the patient cannot be warmed up, and the chilliness is aggravated by the slightest movement. The mouth is dry, the patient extremely irritable and sensitive to the slightest draft.

Influenza

We are all familiar with the signs and symptoms of the flu, which is often epidemic in character and is attributed to viral infection. Influenza usually begins with the symptoms of an upper respiratory ailment and progresses to aches and pains in muscles and joints, often accompanied by a high fever. In the case of flu epidemics, homeopaths will generally discover a remedy epidemicus, or perhaps a few epidemic remedies, that will give relief.

Influenza can progress to seriously complicated conditions, such as pneumonia. In any case that is not responding to treatment and is getting worse, a physician should be consulted.

After contact with someone sick with the flu, homeopaths recommend *Gelsemium* 30, three doses over a twenty-four-hour period, to help prevent infection. If the remedy epidemicus has been determined, the same dosage of that remedy would be used instead of *Gelsemium*.

Once the flu has set in, the following remedies are among those that may prove helpful. They may be given in the 30th potency every four hours, or in the 6th for more prolonged use.

Arsenicum album is given when there is great prostration, with exhaustion after the slightest exertion. The patient is chilly, and he has burning pains that are relieved by heat, except for headache, which is better with cold applications. Streaming eyes and nose. Thirsty for small sips of cold water, which make the symptoms worse.

Bryonia is used when the symptoms are slow to develop. The patient wants to lie perfectly still and be let alone. Irritability and anxiety; if the patient becomes delirious, he talks of business or wants to go home when he is already at home. The patient has internal heat, external coldness, and great thirst for cold drinks. Dry cough, with stitching pains;

the cough may produce headache. Threatened pleurisy. The tongue is coated white. Pains are worse from any movement or from noise, better with pressure on the affected part.

Eupatorium perfoliatum is prescribed when there are severe pains in the limbs and back, with a feeling that the bones are broken and soreness and aching of the bones. There are chills in the spine, bursting, throbbing headaches, and sore eyeballs. Perspiration relieves all symptoms except the headache.

Probably the most commonly indicated remedy in typical symptoms of flu is *Gelsemium*, given when there is irritation in the watery discharge, and much sneezing. The *Gelsemium* patient has chills up and down the spine, a great feeling of heaviness and tiredness, and muscular soreness, with heavy head; and drooping eyelids. There is alternating heat and coldness, no thirst, and a violent, bursting headache. Symptoms are relieved by passing large amounts of urine.

The nux vomica patient's symptoms include extreme chilliness, even in a warm room or when covered, aching limbs and back, and upset stomach. There are dry cough and stuffy nose at night. Better when sitting up, worse on lying down. Nose stuffed up at night. The patient is anxious and irritable.

Pyrogenium is indicated when the following symptom picture appears: Intractable coldness, chill creeping up spine. Bursting headache. Hot stage with profuse sweat that does not reduce temperature. Severe aching pains in back and limbs and in bones. Patient feels beaten and bruised; bed feels too hard. The patient is intensely restless; movement relieves pains. Thumping heartbeat, rapid pulse. Disturbance of relationship between temperature and pulse; high temperature with slow pulse, or vice versa. Patient sleeps deeply, as if comatose.

Rhus toxicodendron is prescribed for the following pattern: The patient feels stiff, lame, and bruised on beginning motion, but pains become better with continued motion, until he becomes weak and must rest. Symptoms are worse in cold, damp weather, or if patient remains damp after perspiring. Aching in bones. Great thirst, with dry tongue, mouth, and throat. Anxiety and fear, worse at night. Restlessness; pains keep the patient moving.

Indigestion

Discomfort arising from disordered digestive functions may vary in severity, and aside from more serious organic causes, may arise from incorrect eating or drinking habits, or from mental tension and anxiety. If severe or persistent symptoms appear in a person who does not usually suffer from indigestion, the cause should be investigated by a physician. Homeopathic remedies for indigestion include the following:

Arsenicum album is frequently employed in cases of food poisoning. *Arsenicum* indigestion is characterized by the following symptoms: Burning pain in the stomach, beginning soon after eating or shortly after midnight, better with warm applications. Distended, painful abdomen, sensitive to touch; feeling of a weight like a stone in the stomach. Patient cannot bear the sight or smell of food. Nausea, retching, vomiting after the slightest quantity of food, leading to weakness and exhaustion with icy coldness. Nausea and vomiting worse between 1:00 A.M. and 3:00 A.M. Thirsty for small amounts at frequent intervals. Cold drinks aggravate symptoms; warm drinks ameliorate.

Bryonia is prescribed when the following symptom picture is present: Pain and pressure in stomach soon after eating. Abdominal pain better with hot applications. Patient lies very still, worse from any disturbance, mental or physical, worse from motion. Nausea and vomiting on raising head and trying to sit. Thirsty for large quantities, but water comes up as soon as it enters the stomach. Vomiting of bile and water immediately after eating or drinking. Indigestion from overeating or from eating rich foods.

Carbo vegetabilis is indicated for the following symptoms: Pain in pit of stomach about half an hour after eating, spreading to chest (heartburn). Even the simplest food disagrees. Acute indigestion after eating pork, rich food, spoiled fish or meat, or especially fatty foods or rancid fats. Great accumulation of gas, with distention of stomach as if it would burst. Food all seems to turn to wind. Much belching and flatulence, which temporarily relieve discomfort. Averse to meat, milk, fat; desire for sweet and salty foods. Heartburn and regurgitation of food. Symptoms produced by gas are better sitting up, worse lying down.

Nux vomica is perhaps the most frequently employed remedy for gastrointestinal disorders. Characteristic nux symptoms include: Disordered stomach, from the ill effects of overindulgence in coffee, tobacco, alcohol, highly seasoned foods, or late hours. The patient may be a chronic user of allopathic medicines for indigestion, which only makes each successive episode worse. Heartburn, bloating, pain in stomach, inclination to vomit. Overeating and improper eating. Sensitivity and irritability. Symptoms are worse from lack of exercise or sleep, alcohol, coffee, tobacco; better with hot foods and fluids, after stool. Nausea and vomiting in the morning. Nux vomica is also an important remedy in cases of food poisoning. Hangover remedy. Desire for fat, beer, brandy; aversion to meat, coffee, water, tobacco.

Pulsatilla is used in gastric disorders from overeating, eating rich food or ice cream, etc. Bloating and feeling of having eaten too much one to two hours after eating. Belching up of rancid food, slimy mouth. Bad taste in mouth. Vomiting of food taken some hours before, especially after emotional stress. Cravings for indigestible or unusual things. Absence of thirst with dry mouth. Restlessness; patient cannot lie still because of gastric and bowel symptoms. Patient is worse in a warm room, from warm or rich food. Better from taking cold things, walking about slowly, fresh air.

4

QUESTIONS AND ANSWERS ABOUT HOMEOPATHIC TREATMENT

WHAT FOODS, BEVERAGES, AND DRUGS MUST I AVOID IF I'M UNDER HOMEOPATHIC TREATMENT?

There is some disagreement among homeopaths when it comes to determining the extent of dietary and other prohibitions. In the *Organon*, Hahnemann gives a long list of substances to be avoided, particularly by patients with chronic diseases: these substances include coffee, Chinese and herb teas, various liquors and highly spiced foods, some vegetables, and cosmetics. Habits such as debauchery, masturbation, reading of obscene books, and overexertion of mind or body are all to be avoided also since they may obstruct the cure.[1] In the case of foods, Hahnemann explains his prohibitions by saying that the substances named may have medicinal effects of their own that can interfere with the action of a remedy.

In more recent times, homeopaths have tended to relax

1. Samuel Hahnemann, *Organon of Medicine*, trans. with Preface by William Boericke, M.D., and Introduction by James Krauss, M.D. (New Delhi: B. Jain Publishers, 1976) footnote to section 260. There are many editions of the *Organon*; all quotations herein will be from the edition cited here.

many of these restrictions, but there remain a few substances that are still believed to antidote the effects of homeopathic remedies. Most prominent and least controversial of these are products containing camphor, along with *all* allopathic medicines. The patient is generally withdrawn from allopathic medications before the homeopath will begin prescribing. There are some exceptions. Some homeopaths will treat an insulin-dependent diabetic if it appears that the insulin will not interfere with the homeopathic remedy; as treatment progresses and the body is stimulated to produce its own insulin, the insulin can gradually be withdrawn. George Vithoulkas notes that it is virtually impossible to treat some patients who have been given large doses of powerful allopathic drugs for long periods of time. Some patients are dependent on cortisone and cannot be safely withdrawn; similarly, patients who have taken antiepileptic medication for many years may suffer almost continuous seizures upon withdrawal of their drugs and therefore cannot be treated homeopathically.

There is some disagreement on the question of coffee drinking. There is a general consensus that coffee antidotes at least some remedies—nux vomica, for example. Vithoulkas says that coffee will eventually antidote any remedy, but that the antidoting effect may take a longer or shorter period of time; for this reason, he tells patients under constitutional treatment that they can never drink coffee, for they will suffer a relapse. Other homeopaths say that coffee does not appear to antidote all remedies, and unless they believe the remedy given is specifically antidoted by coffee, they will permit the patient to keep drinking coffee within reasonable limits. Some patients who have been under homeopathic treatment for years report that they continue to drink coffee and have never had a remedy antidoted.

Since caffeine is generally considered the antidoting substance in coffee, some homeopaths say that it is all right to drink decaffeinated coffee. Others point out that chemicals used in the decaffeination process may have a drug effect of their own.

Of course, black tea also contains caffeine. There is not the same general prohibition among homeopaths against tea drinking, but homeopaths do advise their patients not to drink herb teas, or at least not to drink the same herb tea habitually, since the herb will have a drug effect that may interfere with homeopathic treatment.

Other substances suspected of antidoting remedies include fluoride in toothpaste and anesthetics used in dental operations.

When a patient suffers a relapse, or a return of his original symptoms, the first thing the homeopath will do is inquire closely into the patient's dietary pattern and other habits. Often it will turn out that the patient has done something to antidote the remedy; for example, the patient may have taken it upon himself to use a cortisone ointment for a skin eruption, or he may have drunk coffee or used a camphorated product. Emotional stress can also interfere with the action of remedies. When the antidoting substance is removed or the stressful circumstance corrected, homeopaths report that the remedy can be repeated and its action will hold.

Although Hahnemann imposed many dietary restrictions on patients with chronic diseases, when it came to acute disease. he advised allowing the patient to eat according to her desires. On the other hand, some homeopaths believe that correction of a patient's dietary and drug habits is an absolutely essential element of the homeopathic therapeutic process. Thus Roger Schmidt, M.D., remarked in an interview,

Tobacco, especially, is *out!* . . . Tobacco has a bad effect not only on the remedy, but on the health. So it has to be removed. In the same way, and for the same reasons, you must be very firm about the patient's diet. If you correct it you will already have some good results in a great many cases.[2]

Other homeopathic physicians believe that although measures such as proper diet and exercise may help to bring the patient into the best possible condition at his present level of health, it is only through the action of the correctly selected homeopathic remedy that he can move to an altogether different plane of health, through the removal of the layers

2. "Seminar with Roger A. Schmidt, M.D.," *Homeotherapy* 1, no. 7 (August 1975): p. 6.

of miasms that are impeding the flow of balancing energies within the organism.

Although patients are encouraged to give up injurious habits such as tobacco smoking, excessive alcoholic intake, and the use of "illicit" drugs, homeopaths often find it both necessary and possible to treat people as they are, with all their improper habits. Following a technique popularized by the French homeopath, Gallavardin, Dr. Jack Cooper reports that he was able to change the drinking patterns of numerous chronic alcoholics. The Gallavardin technique, in part, bases the selection of the remedy on the mental symptoms that the alcoholic presents when he is intoxicated: the mean drunk, the happy drunk, the tearful drunk, etc. The remedy is often administered to the patient without his knowledge— added to his food or even to his liquor. Dr. Cooper and others who have treated alcoholics homeopathically observe that the properly selected remedy can actually create an aversion to alcohol, or a change from habitual excessive drinking to normal social drinking patterns. Dr. Bhaghat Singh notes that patients who show real problems with drinking or marijuana smoking may, after homeopathic treatment, no longer be able to stand these drugs.

Homeopathic physicians may differ as to specific dietary and drug prohibitions for their patients, but one thing is universally true: homeopathic treatment is predicated on the patient's accurate reporting of his habits, as well as his pathology. If you do not wish to follow your doctor's instructions on diet and use of alcohol and other drugs, you may find yourself in the uncomfortable position of concealing what you have been doing, which might produce stress and interfere with your treatment. Certainly such inaccurate reporting will not give your doctor a clear picture of why a certain remedy may fail to act. Since health care should be a cooperative effort between you and your physician, it is wise to select a doctor whose advice you respect and can follow. If you disagree with his advice, or feel you cannot follow it, discuss it frankly with him. Only then will you be able to define the limits of what homeopathic treatment can accomplish for you.

CAN HOMEOPATHIC REMEDIES REPLACE ANTIBIOTICS?

The introduction of modern antibiotics was certainly one of the most valuable developments in twentieth-century allopathic medicine. With the use of the sulfa drugs and then penicillin, formerly intractable infectious diseases became susceptible to allopathic treatment. Homeopaths generally welcomed these discoveries as enthusiastically as did allopaths, for many lives were being saved. However, over the years, since the first of these miracle drugs were introduced, we have seen a continuous proliferation of new antibiotics, many of which appear to have even more toxic side effects than penicillin. For example, tetracycline, a widely prescribed broad-spectrum antibiotic, has been noted to produce the following: permanent discoloration and deficient enamel in the teeth of the developing fetus, as well as in the infant and the young child; liver toxicity and biochemical imbalances in the blood of patients with kidney disease; sensitivity of the skin to sunlight; and toxic effects on the fetus, including impaired skeletal development.

Why has there been a need for an ever-increasing number of antibacterial agents, some of which have demonstrable toxic effects? Experience has shown that indiscriminate use of an antibiotic fosters the development of new strains of bacteria that are resistant to the drug; new antibiotics must then be developed to combat these organisms. For example, with the widespread treatment of gonorrhea with antibiotics, new strains of the organism involved, *Neisseria gonorrhoeae*, have developed, and they are not susceptible to the usual antibiotics. Some such cases may resist even the most strenuous treatment, and since gonorrhea has reached epidemic proportions in the United States, the threat of the development of resistant organisms represents a great danger.

When an antibiotic eradicates a certain kind of bacteria in the human organism, other bacteria will thrive in the absence of the microorganisms that held them in balance. George Vithoulkas points out that the use of antibiotics can alter the patient's level of susceptibility, so that he may suffer a succession of infections with ever more intractable bacteria. A patient who has been treated for a *Staphylococcus* infection may subsequently develop an infection with *Proteus* organisms; when this in turn is treated with antibiotics, the patient's susceptibility may move to another level and he may become infected with even more virulent species.

Many broad-spectrum antibiotics destroy beneficial bacteria as well as harmful ones; for example, the bacteria in the intestines are instrumental in the digestion of food and the synthesis of essential vitamins.

Even in allopathic practice, the value of antibiotics is open to serious question. If orthodox physicians had any other way to treat virulent bacterial infections, they would probably avoid the wholesale use of antibiotics, since they know that such use is merely promoting the development of more resistant strains in the long run. If antibiotics could be used selectively, only when there is an urgent need, the accelerating pattern of development of resistant organisms could be held within reasonable limits.

Homeopathic theory holds that proper homeopathic treatment can cure any infectious disease. We have noted that, in the homeopathic view, the presence of bacteria is not the sole cause of disease, but rather the result of a prior disease. In order for bacteria to reproduce to the detriment of the patient's health, there must be a susceptibility on the level of the patient's inner regulatory mechanism; this is why some people exposed to a bacterial infection will get sick and others won't. The properly selected homeopathic remedy is said to remove that inner susceptibility and thereby create an environment that is no longer hospitable to the infecting organism. Sometimes the patient's response to a homeopathic remedy can be spectacularly rapid, as is illustrated in some of the case studies in chapter 7.

Many infectious diseases are self-limited; that is, the patient, provided he has sufficient vitality, will recover in time, no matter what treatment is given. Thus homeopaths will not necessarily intervene in every acute disease, but will sometimes allow the illness to run its course so that the patient can benefit from the immunity he derives from the illness. Childhood diseases are often handled in this manner.

There is no reason to assume that antibiotics are the final answer to the treatment of infectious diseases; they merely happen to be the approach that is proving most effective in allopathic medicine at the present time. The observed side effects, the presence of "allergies" to antibiotics in some individuals, the fostering of resistant organisms, and the eradication of bacteria that are essential to the proper functioning of the body are all signs that antibiotics are not the ultimate weapon against infectious disease. Broad-spectrum antibiotics are widely used today partly because they save time and trouble. The physician can respond quickly in the case of dangerous conditions, and the patient's symptoms will be alleviated, although no one can predict what the long-range effects of the drug will be—for the patient and for the human species as a whole.

Orthodox medicine has shown impressive results in the treatment of bacterial infections, but it has yet to find a "specific" treatment for viral infections. Viruses essentially graft themselves onto body cells in a parasitic relationship, injecting their own DNA into the cells and interfering with the cells' informational content. Therefore, viruses cannot be reached as easily by chemotherapeutic means as can bacteria, for bacteria maintain a discrete identity within the body tissues and fluids. Current research indicates that chemotherapeutic agents being tested against viral disease are highly toxic and may well interfere with essential cellular processes within the human organism. Homeopathy treats viral infections in the same way that it treats bacterial infections, by prescribing on the basis of the Law of Similars, without worrying about what specific etiologic agent is "responsible" for the disease.

The key to the homeopathic treatment of infectious diseases, as of all diseases, lies in proper prescribing. Ideally, the homeopath should never have to resort to the antibiotic drugs of allopathic medicine. If the case is properly taken and the symptoms properly repertorized, the correct remedy should always be able to be found. In practice, however, if the patient is gravely ill, many homeopaths will administer antibiotics if they feel there is not enough time to work out the case and find the proper homeopathic remedy. If the homeopath recognizes that his knowledge is not sufficient to work out the case properly, such a choice will be in the best interests of the patient. Proponents of strict, classical homeopathy deplore this situation and hope that more and more prescribers will master the science of homeopathy on the deepest levels and thus be able to avoid such allopathic treatment in emergencies.

We might add a speculative note. There is widespread concern about the dangers of research in bacteriologic warfare; scientists and laypeople alike portray the possible disastrous consequences of the escape of virulent organisms that have been specifically bred to resist chemotherapy. Mysterious illnesses, such as "legionnaire's disease," have also aroused public interest. The allopathic response to legionnaire's disease was to search for an etiologic agent in order to determine the proper medicine to eradicate the hypothesized "bacteria" responsible. In theory, homeopathic treatment could yield impressive results in such instances for two reasons: (1) both situations have the characteristics of epidemics; hence, a single remedy or group of remedies could be determined for each particular epidemic as the proper treatment in the majority of cases; and (2) since homeopathy selects the remedy on the basis of symptoms alone, identification of the organism involved would not be necessary, nor would it be necessary to develop a chemotherapeutic agent that had the specific effect of eradicating that organism.

Such doomsday thinking is not pleasant. Still, given the scenarios envisioned by the opponents of bacteriologic warfare research, it would appear that homeopathy might offer a possible response to such emergencies.

WHAT CONDITIONS CAN HOMEOPATHY NOT CURE?

We must remember that homeopathy does not treat diseases, it treats people. Because a homeopathic physician has successfully cured a case of cancer with a certain remedy, it does not mean that that remedy is a cure for cancer, nor does it mean that homeopathy can cure all cases of cancer. It simply means that the homeopath, through proper prescribing, has managed to eradicate the complex of miasms that led to the symptomatology of malignant tumor in one particular patient.

We have mentioned that some cases are not suited to homeopathic treatment. Gross trauma often requires surgical intervention (severe lacerations, broken bones, etc.); and there are pathological conditions in which organic change stands in the way of homeopathic treatment, and these can only be treated through surgical intervention. Still, many apparent surgical cases do respond to homeopathic treatment, and if there is not a real emergency, the homeopath may elect to treat a condition with remedies before referring his patient to a surgeon. Acute appendicitis, although usually considered a surgical condition, may respond to proper prescribing. In China, herbs are used in treating appendicitis, with a 90 percent cure rate, as stated in a recent National Academy of Science report. In the case of gallstones or kidney stones, homeopaths observe that the proper remedy can produce changes in the chemical composition of body fluids, so that the stones dissolve or are crushed.

There are some cases that homeopaths generally consider incurable. The disease process may be too far advanced for homeopathic remedies to do more than provide palliation. By watching the direction and progress of symptoms after administration of a remedy, the homeopath will be able to determine the prognosis of such cases. In a case where there is deep pathology, when the patient experiences a short amelioration followed by an aggravation, the homeopath may suspect that the case is incurable and open only to palliation with the remedy that is called for with each successive relapse.

Some cases have been so complicated by allopathic drugging that the patient cannot be withdrawn from the drugs without suffering a profound and potentially fatal aggravation (or reappearance) of symptoms that have been suppressed for years. Homeopaths will generally tell such drug-dependent patients that homeopathic treatment cannot help them.

Another kind of illness that may be homeopathically incurable is the serious psychotic case, in which the patient has been on antipsychotic medications for a number of years. Although George Vithoulkas reports success in a few such cases in which he reluctantly undertook treatment, he generally advises homeopaths not to accept such long-standing psychotic cases.

Some cases have been so badly mixed up by improper homeopathic drugging that the homeopathic physician can no longer sort out the symptoms on which to prescribe, for the patient is presenting the symptoms of the remedies he has been given in the past. Such cases can be even more frustrating for the homeopath than those complicated by allopathic drugging, for the improper administration of the homeopathic remedies has "permanently" interfered with the expressions of the vital force that are the only clue to correct prescribing. In allopathic drugging, once the drugs are discontinued, the patient's symptoms will become relatively clear. The homeopath's drugs are highly reactive and should be avoided by the unskilled prescriber.

Homeopathic physicians probably see a disproportionate number of difficult, complicated, and incurable cases because patients often do not go to a homeopath until they have exhausted a number of other possible medical approaches. Homeopaths are frequently confronted with cases complicated by overdrugging, multiple surgeries, and dependence on allopathic medication. That homeopathic physicians are able to unravel some such cases and afford relief to patients is a testimony to the effectiveness of such treatment.

Homeopaths also feel that their approach is the most appropriate in so-called terminal cases, where the pathology is far advanced and the patient apparently declining toward death. Rather than force the patient to pass his last days in a narcotized mental state or in discomfort from last-ditch rounds of radiation, surgery, chemotherapy, and other drastic measures, the homeopath may be able to afford palliation of the patient's pains and leave his mind clear as he reaches the end. Although some homeopaths allude to the use of remedies to produce euthanasia, George Vithoulkas reports that many apparently terminal patients have survived for years under palliative homeopathic treatment.

CAN HOMEOPATHIC TREATMENT BE DANGEROUS?

Any form of medicine can be dangerous in inexpert hands. There are two classes of dangers in medical practice: those arising from things that are left undone, and those arising from things that are done. Like any physician, the homeopath must have a solid background in anatomy, physiology, and the natural history of diseases, as well as having extensive clinical experience. Dangerous omissions in homeopathic practice might include failure to recognize a case that clearly calls for surgical intervention. A prescriber with limited knowledge of homeopathic principles might similarly endanger his patient if he failed to recognize his own limitations and neglected to consult a more experienced homeopath or to use other measures that will be more certain of putting the patient out of immediate danger.

There has been a recent trend for allopathic treatment to be enforced by law in certain kinds of illnesses. Parents who have opted for alternatives to insulin therapy in diabetes or chemotherapy in childhood leukemia have been threatened with having their children taken out of their custody. Court battles over who has the right to order the discontinuance of artificial life support have brought such medicolegal questions before the public eye. Patients of homeopathic physicians may find themselves involved in medicolegal battles, as do Christian Scientists, Jehovah's Witnesses, patients of naturopaths, and others who for philosophical, religious, or scientific reasons opt for nonorthodox approaches to healing. It is always the physician's responsibility to advise the patient of the risks involved in electing an alternative to prescribed allopathic treatment; however, even more dangerous is the encroachment by government upon the patient's right to freedom of choice.

In the course of proper homeopathic treatment, the patient

may pass through dangerous crises, and the physician must be extremely alert for signs of developments that threaten the patient's life. Withdrawing a patient from allopathic drugs can present dangers, and the homeopath must be thoroughly versed in the possible consequences of such withdrawal before advising the patient to discontinue any drugs to "clear" himself for homeopathic treatment.

Although homeopathic remedies are given in very small, even immaterial doses, clinical experience has demonstrated that they can have profoundly disturbing effects on the patient's economy. In cases with deep physical pathology, the administration of a high-potency homeopathic remedy may produce such a profound aggravation that a patient with insufficient vitality might not survive the crisis. For this reason, homeopaths generally restrict their prescribing to the low potencies in cases of advanced and deep physical pathology. In cases with serious and prolonged aggravations with no subsequent amelioration, Kent advises that the remedy may need to be antidoted and that the patient is probably incurable. Vithoulkas, on the other hand, believes that the physician must be alert for changes in symptoms calling for a change of remedy; he says that as soon as the picture of a second remedy is clear, it should be given immediately, and the case may eventually progress to a cure.

Another danger can arise from the direction of cure. According to Hering's law, symptoms will disappear first from more important and then from less important organs, from the center toward the periphery, from above downwards, and in the reverse order of their appearance. If we assume that deep-seated mental problems are at the innermost level of the patient's symptom complex, then in the course of treatment mental symptoms may disappear and symptoms may begin to appear on the physical plane. For example, a patient complaining primarily of mental problems may also have a history of a heart condition, which has become quiescent during the time of severe mental symptoms. As the patient's mental symptoms begin to disappear under constitutional treatment, the symptoms may move to the physical plane and the patient may have a heart infarct. With scrupulous attention to correct prescribing, particularly avoiding the high potencies, the homeopath can help the patient through such healing crises, but a mistake on the part of the physician can be fatal. Yet Vithoulkas observes that he has seen over thirty thousand cases and has never seen a case in which the movement of the symptoms from the mental sphere into the physical body proved fatal; it is as if the inner regulatory mechanism determines a channel through which symptoms can regress without killing the patient.

As we have mentioned, the homeopathic prescriber must also be aware of the dangers of prescribing certain remedies too often or too high, since such incorrect prescribing can implant a drug disease that will be extremely difficult to clear up.

Many popularizers of homeopathy claim that it is "harmless" or completely "safe." Any form of treatment that can effect profound changes in the human organism must be approached with care, for it is a double-edged sword. Kent makes this abundantly clear in his admonition to students of homeopathy:

If our medicines were not powerful enough to kill folks, they would not be powerful enough to cure sick folks. It is well for you to realize that you are dealing with razors when dealing with high potencies. . . . They are means of tremendous harm as well as of tremendous good.[3]

ARE THERE SUBSTANCES IN OUR ENVIRONMENT THAT MAY ACT AS POTENTIZED DRUGS?

The answer to this question, of course, is yes. According to the homeopathic view, the contaminants in our environment may be having a profoundly deleterious effect on the health of entire nations.

The fluoridation of our drinking water is universally opposed by homeopaths for the obvious reason that the fluoride, dissolved and dispersed in our water supply and then subjected to succession as it flows through pipes and is alter-

3. James Tyler Kent, A.M., M.D., *Lectures on Homeopathic Materia Medica* (New Delhi: Jain Publishing Co., 1972), p. 577.

nately stopped and released by valves, is being subjected to a process of potentization. Dr. Bhaghat Singh observes that in New York City thousands of people are suffering from the effects of fluoride in their water; he sees many patients presenting the mental symptoms of fluoric acid provings. When he treats such people with *Fluoricum acidum* in the IM 1,000th potency, he reports that they return to more balanced functioning. In order to eliminate the effects of potentized fluorides in our drinking water, Dr. Singh says that the water must be boiled; potentized remedies have been shown to lose their power when exposed to high temperatures.

Of course, in addition to the deliberate contamination of our environment, as in the case of fluoridation, industrial processes are filling our atmosphere, our soil, our water, and ultimately our bodies with innumerable other chemicals that may also be acting as potentized drugs and implanting drug diseases in us. Patients exposed on a daily basis to automobile exhaust have been treated with potencies of sulfuric acid, one of the components of such exhaust, and good results have been obtained.

Another important source of potentized toxins is our food. The use of additives, insecticides, and herbicides; the presence of chemical waste in our water supply; and the deliberate addition of hormones and other chemicals to the feed of animals may lead to the potentization of these substances through the biological processes of the animal or plant that depends on the feed, water, or soil as a food source. Once the toxin has been subjected to the metabolic processes of the organism that has ingested it, it may become incorporated into the organism's tissues in potentized form. We are just beginning to become aware of the dangers of this process, as in such diverse cases as the presence of stilbestrol in our beef, mercury (from industrial waste) in seafood, and strontium 90 in milk from cows who have fed on grass contaminated by radioactive fallout.

When the symptom picture of the offending substance is clear, homeopathy treats the symptoms arising from such contamination either by giving a high potency of the toxic substance or by giving an antidoting remedy. With the multiplicity of toxins in our environment, the pictures of such poisoning are becoming more and more complex, and we can only hope that all possible efforts will be made to reduce such contaminants before incurable drug diseases have been implanted upon all of humanity.

IS THE PATIENT'S RESPONSE TO A HOMEOPATHIC REMEDY JUST A PLACEBO EFFECT?

The word *placebo* is derived from the Latin verb meaning "to please." A placebo, as used in medicine, is a physiologically inert substance, such as a sugar pill, whose purpose is to please, or placate, the patient. The placebo is widely used as a control in the experimental evaluation of the action of new drugs.

Because homeopathic remedies are prepared in immaterial doses and administered on sugar pills, critics have consistently claimed that any observed effects on the patient must be the result of suggestion, or the placebo effect.

Homeopaths, when confronted with this argument, conventionally adduce the evidence of successful homeopathic treatment of infants and animals. In both cases the influence of suggestion is highly unlikely, but the issue of the placebo is a searching philosophical question whose exploration might shed additional light on the homeopathic approach, for homeopaths do make conscious use of the placebo effect in treating their patients.

In order to secure the patient's cooperation, unmedicated powders or sugar pills may be given at two critical stages: (1) at the beginning of the case, if the homeopath needs more time to work out the proper remedy but wants the patient to refrain from using other medications; and (2) when the remedy has begun to act and the homeopath wants to prevent the patient from interfering with its action.

Furthermore, homeopaths acknowledge that there may be a distinct placebo benefit in the therapeutic setting itself. The homeopath's detailed attention to the patient's complaints and his focus on the individual as a distinct, whole person often have obvious psychological benefit, especially when contrasted with the impersonal setting of the usual allopathic interview and examination. Even allopathic practitioners realize that the very fact that the patient appears in the office and entrusts his health care to the doctor establishes a therapeutic set that may promote recovery independently of any treatment that is given.

Placebo might be the single greatest medicine ever discovered within the healing arts. What it does is reach directly to the self-healing, reactive inner regulatory mechanisms of the human organism and stimulate a return to equilibrium. The mechanisms at work appear to be largely unconscious. The information conveyed by the placebo is "heal yourself," and amazingly, the patient often responds by doing just that.

In a recent book, Norman Cousins surveys some of the new evidence of the breadth and depth of the action of the placebo.[4] Under the proper experimental conditions, with the proper expectations aroused in the subjects, placebo can have amazingly specific effects—for example, the reduction of the amount of fat and protein in the blood, changes in the numbers of certain specialized blood cells, relief of arthritic pains, prevention of withdrawal symptoms in morphine addicts, and relief from bleeding ulcers. Moreover, subjects in placebo studies may experience not only the specific desired action of the drug they think they have been given, but also the accompanying side effects.

Such findings confirm Hahnemann's premise of the existence of the reactive vital force—an energy field which, given the proper stimulation, can restore equilibrium on the physical, emotional, and mental planes of the patient. According to the homeopathic analysis, in an ideal state of health the vital force would always be able to cure its own imbalances, but because the human economy has been distorted by chronic miasms, the channels through which the self-healing energies flow have been selectively blocked. Such blockage has, in each individual at any given time, a characteristic pattern, manifested in perceptible alterations in the

4. Norman Cousins, *Anatomy of an Illness as Perceived by the Patient* (New York: W. W. Norton & Co., 1979), pp. 49–71.

patient's mental, physical, and emotional functions and in gross physical pathology—all of which are taken as symptoms. The homeopath selects a remedy that is capable of producing in healthy individuals the same symptoms that the patient is suffering from. The informational content of such a remedy is thus more specific than the "heal yourself" of the placebo; through the transient aggravation of the patient's symptoms by the *simillimum*, the vital force is shown the pathways along which it must act in order to restore equilibrium.

Carefully observed provings of homeopathic remedies have shown that the high potencies are capable of eliciting specific, predictable symptoms that distinguish them from placebo. In homeopathic practice, observed homeopathic aggravations followed by recovery also suggest that the potentized remedy is more specific in its action than the placebo. Patients may experience an aggravation regardless of whether or not they have been warned by the doctor that such an aggravation may occur. If the remedy were merely acting as a placebo, it would seem more likely that the patient would experience immediate relief, without an aggravation.

Contemporary studies of the placebo phenomenon constitute the strongest evidence we have for the existence of the nonmaterial mechanism that Hahnemann called the vital force. Now that the existence of this nonphysical energetic mechanism has been demonstrated in allopathic research laboratories, the time may be ripe for scientists to reexamine their notions as to whether potentized medicines might also be able to act on a nonphysical level.

5

IS HOMEOPATHY SCIENTIFIC?

SCIENTIFIC TOOLS IN MEDICINE

Because homeopathy is so different from the kind of medicine we are used to, it might appear that it is not as "scientific" as modern orthodox medicine. Living as we do in a highly technological age, we may feel suspicious of a therapeutic approach that does not make full use of the potentially beneficial tools of modern science.

As science has developed, orthodox medicine has borrowed heavily from its discoveries and applied them to diagnostic and therapeutic procedures. In arriving at a diagnosis, the contemporary allopathic physician makes use of the sciences of chemistry, optics, microbiology, and physics. All these objective parameters yield data that are used to determine the disease from which the patient suffers.

In reality, few if any patients correspond in their illnesses to the groupings of objective data that define such disease entities. Diagnostic categories merely represent a statistical averaging of measurable parameters observed in large groupings of patients; and such averages do not take into consideration the many individualizing factors that will determine the patient's response to the therapy prescribed for a particular disease entity.

Diagnostic names are not needed in homeopathy. If a disease is given a name (other than for the purposes of record keeping or explaining the condition to the patient and his family), it is *named for the remedy that will cure it.* Such terminology may sound strange to the allopathically

115

conditioned ear, but even among allopaths there is a growing recognition that too-broad diagnostic categories can lead to the employment of drugs that have undesirable side effects. Two eminent psychopharmacologists, Abraham Hoffer and Humphry Osmond, have proposed that researchers look for drugs with specific actions and then discover the conditions that will respond to such drugs: "The essence of this method is to find the clinical situation which will respond to a known chemical."[1] In the context of such contemporary statements, it does not seem so peculiar to talk about a *"Pulsatilla* illness" or a *"Lycopodium* patient."

Underlying modern allopathic therapeutics is an ancient tradition summed up in the Latin phrase *tolle causam*, or "remove the cause." Of course all therapy has this goal, but allopathy believes that the cause must be identified in order to determine the proper treatment—thus, theory must precede practice. Allopathy has impressive theories to explain the causes of many diseases, yet these theories are continually changing, and as they change, the therapy based on each theoretical model is discarded in favor of a new approach.

Homeopathy is not particularly concerned with identifying the causes of disease, for treatment depends only on the similarity of the diseased state to a medicine that will produce the same symptoms in healthy persons. Homeopathy is a set of principles for the application of medicines in the treatment of illness. These principles have remained stable over 170 years of practice, and the structure of the homeopathic doctrine is such that new information can continually be incorporated into the existing body of knowledge. As new drugs are proved and added to the materia medica, they can be applied according to the same principles that guided homeopathic prescribing in Hahnemann's time.

The allopathic explanation of disease in terms of the very latest theoretical models does not in itself make allopathy more scientific; such models have scientific value only if

1. Abraham Hoffer and Humphry Osmond, "Double-Blind Clinical Trials," *Journal of Neuropsychiatry* 2 (1961): 222, quoted in Harris Coulter, *Homeopathic Medicine* (Washington, D.C.: American Foundation of Homeopathy, 1972), p. 60, note.

they prove to have some stability when tested against experience.

In actual treatment, the orthodox physician again has recourse to the products of modern science. He may use radiation to destroy unwanted tissue, or he may use a drug that has been shown to alter a specific biochemical function in animals. In modern pharmacology, there is great emphasis on "structure-activity relationships"—the prediction or explanation of drug action on the basis of the molecular configuration of the compound in question. Here again the principle of "remove the cause" influences orthodox therapeutics, for the allopath wants to know *why* a drug has a particular effect and tends to be suspicious of any drug for which such an explanation, no matter how faulty, is lacking.

The homeopath is not concerned with theoretical explanations of drug action; he bases his prescribing solely on actual observation of the effects of his medicines on healthy human beings. Such observations define the range of the action of the medicine and provide all the information needed to help select the proper remedy for a given patient.

How does a physician determine whether his patient is getting better or worse? The allopath will repeat the diagnostic tests that told him what disease the patient had at the beginning of treatment; he may also perform additional tests to ascertain whether the drugs he has prescribed have had an adverse effect on other functions. On the basis of X rays, laboratory findings, and clinical examination, the orthodox physician determines whether the patient is showing a return to normal function. Thus the criteria for recovery are largely objective, quantified findings at the physical and functional levels of the patient.

Although the homeopath may similarly review the laboratory values and other objective findings in following the patient, he will also place great importance on how the patient feels, as a whole, in himself. This state of well-being is not something that can be quantified, and so it is often a missing element in the allopathic picture of the patient. Allopathic therapy will persist in the indicated treatment until the patient's laboratory values have returned to an arbitrarily defined normal range. The homeopath places greater value on the patient's report of his own sense of well-being.

According to the homeopathic model of the human organism, the most vital, innermost part of man is reflected precisely by this general feeling of health. Just as we often feel a generalized, vague malaise before we become ill with an acute disease, so is the vital force itself the first part of the organism that is reached by a deep-acting homeopathic remedy. According to Hering's law, as the imbalance in the vital force is resolved at the deepest level, the disease moves outward, manifesting itself in temporary disturbances in the physical sphere and moving from more important to less important organs.

Thus Hering's law gives the homeopath a criterion for monitoring the progress of a case, for it evaluates the patient as a whole and assigns laboratory values, mental state, physical pathology, and functional symptoms their relative importances according to a hierarchical model of the organism. Laboratory values may return to normal, but the patient may not be cured; or, laboratory values may remain slightly beyond the normal range, and the patient may be cured.

One of the reasons modern orthodox medicine appears to be scientific is that it makes use of precise measurements. As we have seen, pathologic and biochemical data are used in the process of diagnosis and hence in determining the nature of the treatment; they are also used to follow the patient's progress and determine the prognosis of the case.

Pathological findings can also be critical in helping the homeopath avoid problems in the course of treatment. The homeopath can make use of modern scientific tools to determine the degree of physical pathology, thus being guided in the selection of the proper remedy and the proper potency so that he will be able to avoid stirring up the vital force in a patient with marked tissue changes. Laboratory findings can also yield pathological data that have the weight of symptoms for the homeopath. X rays and tests of biochemical functions may reveal the site of a problem—for example, internal bleeding—that will guide the homeopath to a remedy that not only produces the external manifestations of the condition, but also has an affinity for the organ involved. As any other doctor, the homeopath makes use of all the tools at his disposal to ensure that the patient is receiving the best and safest treatment he can give.

The contrast between homeopathy and allopathy can be summed up as a difference in the thought processes involved. We shall now examine how the raw data of experience are studied in an orderly way to build up a system of scientific therapeutics in homeopathy.

THE INDUCTIVE METHOD

Anyone who has studied high school science is familiar with the idea of the *inductive* experimental method. This orderly procedure for discovering the laws of nature traces its origins to the writings of the great empiricist Francis Bacon (1561–1626), and it has since evolved into a model for proper scientific inquiry in many fields of human knowledge.

Briefly stated, the inductive method involves three steps: observation, hypothesis, and experimentation. The scientist first observes the world around him and notes that certain phenomena seem to proceed in an orderly manner. On the basis of such observation, he formulates a hypothesis about how such phenomena will act under certain conditions, and he then subjects his hypothesis to an experiment to see whether the predicted phenomena actually occur. The inductive method is based on *experience*; because it proceeds from empirical fact, it always reflects the world as it really is.

In contrast, the *deductive* model, as employed by Aristotle, proceeds from abstract axioms through mathematically rigid logical steps to conclusions about empirical phenomena. The Aristotelian model, in the form of the teachings of Galen, the second-century Greek physician, dominated orthodox medical thought all the way up through the nineteenth century. Because it proceeded from abstract theory, it was extremely resistant to the evidence of experience and was a major factor in orthodox medicine's refusal to acknowledge the correctness of such revolutionary discoveries as the circulation of the blood and the proper delineation of the human anatomy.

In what ways does homeopathy conform to the inductive model? When Hahnemann administered cinchona bark to himself and observed its effects, he noted that the symptoms produced by the drug were similar to those of the disease in which cinchona was curative. He then proceeded to formulate a hypothesis: that the curative power of a drug lies in its ability to produce symptoms similar to those it is used to treat. This hypothesis led to experiments along two different lines. In drug provings, Hahnemann and his associates took other drugs in use during that time to see what symptoms were produced and whether these symptoms were similar to the diseased states in which the drugs were employed. In therapeutic practice, they administered drugs to patients on the basis of similarity and observed whether these drugs were curative. In both provings and practice, the homeopaths reported confirmation of the Law of Similars. For Hahnemann and his followers, it was not necessary to understand why the drugs acted the way they did; if their experience verified that the drugs did act on the principle of similarity, that is all they hoped to know, and they were guided in their practice by the continually accumulating body of evidence in support of this hypothesis. Homeopathic practice, when successful in curing diseased states, yields evidence that the Law of Similars is correct.

The proper application of the scientific method in homeopathy resolves into three phases: (1) provings of remedies; (2) taking the case; and (3) matching the patient's symptoms to those of the proper remedy.

Steps 2 and 3 are best elucidated by illustration. Chapter 7 contains a number of case studies that show how the homeopathic physician elicits symptoms from the patient, what kinds of symptoms he attaches importance to, and how he determines the proper remedy.

Step 1, the proving of drugs, can be reduced to an orderly experimental procedure. Since drug provings are an excellent illustration of the scientific approach in homeopathy, let us examine the methods employed in such provings.

DRUG PROVINGS

In Hahnemann's time, drug provings were conducted in a manner that lacked the rigor of modern experimental studies. The subject took a drug, either in crude or potentized form, and all the symptoms he experienced were recorded. In this way a huge body of symptoms was amassed for each drug, and these complex symptom pictures were then used as the basis for selecting the most similar remedy in diseased states. When a drug prescribed on the basis of similarity cured a particular symptom or group of symptoms, this clinical experience not only provided further verification of the Law of Similars, it also verified the symptom as it had shown itself in the provings. Many of the strange, rare, and peculiar symptoms elicited in only a few provers have been verified over and over in clinical practice when these symptoms have guided the physician to the selection of a curative remedy.

Since Hahnemann's time, there has been considerable refinement of the techniques of drug provings. In order to be sure that the symptoms experienced are the effect of the drug, the following conditions should be met: (1) the person proving the drug should not know what drug he is taking; (2) some provers should be given an inert substance, or placebo, so that the effect of the placebo can be compared with the effect of the drug; and (3) even the person conducting the experiment should not be aware of what drug is being given, or who gets placebo and who gets the drug, so that the experimenter cannot give any signals to the subjects. Studies conforming to these requirements are known as *double-blind provings*.

What does the prover experience after taking a homeopathic remedy? The following excerpted material from Kent's writings describes the effects of a very high potency on a single prover. Kent introduces the prover's own written account with some comments on the circumstances and on the value of the proving:

A proving that was made under my own eye, under the proper rules for proving, demonstrated most clearly that real symptoms were produced by the 10 millionth potency of Lachesis. I had heretofore not believed it possible to procure symptoms from this potency. The prover did not know what the dose was that she took. She brought out one symptom as perfectly new, and it might be doubted as a genuine Lachesis symptom, but the fact that I had discovered the symptom several years before clinically, and confirmed it and verified. Such a symptom the prover did bring out; and such a symptom known to belong to the drug, and that in the very high numbers, removed all doubt in my mind of the possibility of procuring symptoms in such high numbers.

This prover was not in perfect health, I am willing to say in answer to the proper question. She was a very nervous person, extremely sensitive, and a subject of many nervous symptoms. This must of course greatly impair the value of the proving in the eyes of many. A singular fact that I want fully stated here, is, the symptoms of the prover were entirely new and ran their course as an acute miasm should have done, completely subduing all the symptoms peculiar to the prover (with exceptions mentioned), and when the proving or drug symptoms departed, all her old symptoms came back. This shows that she was not proving a similar, that it was not a Homoeopathic aggravation, but that it was a genuine proving. . . . It may be gleaned that a proving may suppress a given sickness. That is just what happened in this most wonderful proving, and is just what happens in some of our best provings. . . .

Another grand lesson is found in the proving, viz; that highly dynamized medicines are capable of suppressing the symptoms of natural diseases, and implanting themselves instead. Another warning to the beginner, that he may not be too hasty in giving medicine to sensitive, nervous patients.

In presenting this proving, as it comes from the pen of the prover, it is my purpose only to say for it, it must stand or fall on its own worth as a proving made to throw light on the great pathogenesis of Lachesis.

Mrs. H.W.A.—Proving of Lachesis 10m. Beginning February 14, 1887. A very nervous little woman who has never been very sick, but always very sensitive to surrounding atmosphere, so that she proves every thing she breathes.

February 14th—Took a few pellets dry on the tongue, 1:30 p.m. Head felt better in a little while. Soon felt a severe, heavy ache in both thighs as though they would come off or break. Slight amelioration by morning. Felt warm blood circulating in legs and feet;

from knees down, are usually cold. Felt happy and jolly, in spite of severe aching. Could not stand as usual during shopping. Upper arms began to ache, 3 p.m., left worst. Pain in legs diminished, as pain in arms increased; could not carry a small parcel. Left arm *aggravated* by hanging. Left arm *ameliorated* by resting in coat. Aching moved upward to the shoulder, as though arm would drop out. Aching extending under scapula. Subsided into an *uneasy* ache after 5 p.m. Weight diminished. Was told I look *pale*. During evening had to rest the *left* leg on chair, and take off the shoe. Elevation relieved the leg, but *left* arm began to ache. Aching pain again went under scapula and *posterior left lung*. Could not lie on right side because of drawing sensation around the heart. Lying on left side *agg*. pain in arm, shoulder, lung and heart. Wondered if I would have heart disease, as my mother died of atrophy of the heart. Restless and suffocated all night.

February 16th—Could not study or give due attention. Heart ached and would stop breath as though it would palpitate, but it did not. Went to sleep that night listening to the beating in head and ears synchronous with heart beat.

February 17th—Aching of entire left side from crest of illium to first rib. Aching under both scapulae, *left* the worse. Upper arm so heavy could hardly raise it. Sensation in arm as if it were pulled. Intense aching between heart and scapulae, and was afraid to stir or breathe, and would raise and lower the shoulder to get relief. Slight palpitation and pain in apex.

February 18th—Pain in apex followed by palpitation. Afraid some one would see and speak of the anxiety. Could hardly hold anything, would slip out of my hands. Feared the increasing palpitation which aroused me frequently in the night. Dreamed of riding in a strong wind which took my breath. Dreamed of riding on horseback. Going swiftly through the air gave me a sinking feeling in the stomach and left thorax. Waked holding my breath. Desire to unfasten dress from sternum to waist line. Could not study in evening, hated everything, books, paper, pencil, lectures; and medicine. Felt like squirming; has often come on since I began taking the drug. Afraid to go to sleep after retiring; put hand on heart to watch its beating. Could rest comfortably upon *left* side, with hand upon heart; so slept. . . .

March 22nd—Slept well; *dreams natural. Dreamed* that on preparing for lectures, could not hurry. There was much soreness and gone feeling in the stomach. Back of head ached. No motion of bowels. First evacuation of urine, thick, deep orange color; unsatisfied feeling, causing burning and smarting of parts. Cold from knees down, ankle aches. But little of the burning and smarting, sensation (scalded) of mouth and stomach, present yesterday A.M.; bloody mucus from left lung. Weak in attempting to walk. Yesterday, while standing for the first time at foot of bed, felt very tall and bed looked small. Felt three feet taller than usual. Toast, raw oysters and "cambric tea" seem to suit. Crave sour things, which for two years have *agg.* my bowels, so also salt. Blisters in mouth, on lips, under nose, disappearing. As eager as a thirsty child for a glass of water. Small moulded stool covered with mucus; feel better.

March 26th—Mournful, dreamy state of mind, as though something very sad were transpiring, took Lach., 9m. . . .

April 6th—Itching in roof of mouth and base of tongue; must rub it. At times burning and pricking on the edge of tongue, *agg.* by smell of tobacco or turpentine. All one feeling in stomach *amel.* by eating. Slow urination, especially after waiting. Sweat middle of night, or after first sleep. Throat feels full. Mouth feels sore. *Agg.* of the burning in mouth and stomach by salt. Dyspnoea *agg.* by slightest exertion. Constriction of the throat, as if something tight were about it. Coughing at night caused by itching in left side of throat, extending to ear. *Amel.* by warmth of hand. Hands puffy and often very warm. Sweat followed by chill (caused by dampness of clothes); then heat, then sleep. Fourth toe joint sore upon under side. Moved to first toe and thought it would be a bunion. So sleepy at 8 p.m. am obliged to retire. Right foot and leg feels large, warm and heavy. Left foot and leg feels small, numb and cold. Quivering in both ears when lying down at night, at times relieved by changes of position. Aching back of both ears. Aching a little above the apex of heart. Throbbing in left side. Slight pain in left ovarian region, sometimes both sides, and then in hypogastrium. During past two weeks swelling induration and smarting of the ducts of sublingual glands. Relieved. Feeling of prolapsed rectum, only relieved by lying on the stomach. Top of head sore and hot. Throat burns and feels raw. Lungs dry and tight. No expectoration after long coughing. Burning smarting with itching.

April 7th—Constipation; feces hard, bleeding from rectum. Feels like cut after stool. Bearing down in rectum, long time after evacuation. Gray spots drop in front of left eye while reading. Caused blur and nervousness. *Agg.* by looking to the left. *Amel.* by continuing to read. Mouth sore; herpes, lower lip, right side. . . .

April 12th—Extreme pleasure causes trembling and twitching for hours, more than would severe fright or sudden surprise. That and mental exertion caused wakefulness until midnight. Waked very early. Annoyed by sudden loss of subject of sentence, in attempts to speak. Effort to hold an idea until it can be expressed. Expression or the real effort, drives subject matter quite out of mind. Aching in occiput, extending to cervical vertebrae. Same pain extending down the arm when walking or upon receiving a jar.[2]

Modern provings of homeopathic remedies can yield impressive evidence of what these medicines can do, and modern provings can confirm the validity and consistency of the symptom images reported by early provers. Moreover, carefully controlled double-blind provings might yield evidence on the more controversial issue of ultramolecular doses. If several provers take a remedy in the 30th potency, let us say, and experience some of the same symptoms that have been associated with that remedy through some 170 years of homeopathic literature, the experiment will suggest that potentized remedies, where not even one molecule of the original drug may be present, might produce predictable effects in the human organism. Since the question of high potencies has been one of the most vexing in the history of homeopathy, such experiments would seem to be sorely needed to establish the scientific respectability of homeopathy in the modern world.

Carefully controlled drug provings are extremely arduous and time-consuming. Each subject must undergo the same sort of interview that is performed in the initial examination of a patient. The experimenter must spend an hour or more taking a complete inventory of the prover's symptoms before the drug is given, so that such symptoms will not be attributed to the action of the drug. As the experiment progresses, the experimentor must perform detailed interviews of the prover to elicit all the symptoms that have appeared since the administration of the drug; to aid this process, the prover keeps a daily written record of his symptoms. In modern allopathic medicine, such an experiment would be easier, since there are virtually unlimited funds and professional personnel available for research. In homeopathy, unfortunately, the number of people qualified to perform such interviews is extremely limited.

The research procedure defined by the American Acad-

2. J. T. Kent, A.M., M.D., *New Remedies, Clinical Cases, Lesser Writings, Aphorisms and Precepts* (New Delhi: B. Jain Publishers, 1976), pp. 429–442.

emy of Homeotherapeutics, a division of the American Institute of Homeopathy, requires that double-blind provings be conducted on any new substance before it can be included in the U.S. Homeopathic Pharmacopoeia. The same procedure could be used to complete the symptom pictures of remedies that were not fully proved in the past. Many early provers stressed the physical symptoms they experienced, paying less attention to the mentals. Some remedies, such as some of the nosodes, are of relatively recent introduction and have never been thoroughly proved. Aside from the obvious educational value of participating in provings, there is still much valuable information to be gained, and there has been some rebirth of interest in homeopathic provings.

Recently a study group in Berkeley, California, conducted a double-blind proving as a step toward defining a method that would be useful for future provings. One member of the group was selected as the proving conductor, and she made up the medicines in numbered packages, some packages containing placebo and some the remedy. Only the conductor of the proving knew what the remedy was, and which package numbers corresponded to placebo. The conductor then withdrew from the experiment, and the provers distributed the packages among themselves and took the contents, one dose a day, in the sequence indicated. For the first week or so, all the provers, unknown to themselves, received placebo. Some continued to receive placebo throughout the proving, and the others, after the period on placebo, took one dose of *Pulsatilla* 30 per day for thirty days.

Because the provers were all students or practitioners of homeopathy, they were able to keep written records of their own symptoms, thus eliminating the need for a trained homeopath to take the symptoms of each prover. Randy Neustaedter, a lay homeopath at Berkeley's Hering Clinic, was one of the provers. He reported his experience as follows:

We developed symptoms. One of the provers developed an ulcer on his cornea, and I developed a very characteristic state which involved mostly cold symptoms, but mental symptoms too, and from the symptoms and their modalities I deduced what the medicine was. . . . I can't remember how long it really took, but I know I didn't go through the month. I stopped the proving, because the symptoms got too severe to continue. They were physical, mostly—a cough, really bad congestion. And the mental state too. And everytime I would go out in the open air it would get better, and I'd come back in and it would get worse again. I had very characteristic symptoms. So I think the proving was a success.

Such were the results after taking a remedy diluted in the proportion of 1:1,000,000,000,000,000,000,000,000,000,000,000,000!

Anyone can prove a medicine. As people become more interested in homeopathy, it is reasonable for them to want to experience the pure effects of a remedy when they are healthy, as a confirmation of one of the basic assumptions of the homeopathic doctrine. Although provings are said to have a beneficial, tonic effect on a healthy person, it is obviously advisable to seek the guidance of an experienced homeopath before undertaking such an experiment.

LABORATORY INVESTIGATIONS OF THE HIGH POTENCIES

Much of the skepticism about homeopathy revolves around the issue of whether the homeopathic potencies can actually produce an effect on the human organism. According to Avogadro's law, beyond the 12th centesimal or the 24th decimal potency it is unlikely that a single molecule of the original medicinal substance will be present in any dose administered to the patient, yet homeopaths report significant effects from potencies as high as the millions! In the reports of provings, evidence of the activity of these very high potencies appears even when the identity of the substance is unknown to the provers, who experienced symptoms characteristic of that substance as recorded in the materia medica.

How do homeopaths account for the activity of the ultramolecular dose? If none of the original remedy is present in material form, the characteristic symptom patterns developed in patients cannot be a result of physiologic action. From Hahnemann on, homeopaths have said that the remedies contain a pattern that, because of its similarity to the pattern of distortion of the vital force, removes the patient's symptoms on the basis of like cures like. With the recent refinement of the physical sciences, we can come closer to speculating about the realm in which this pattern might lie.

Modern attempts to account for the activity of the high potencies have taken their cue from such branches of contemporary science as quantum chemistry. Barnard and Stephenson in a 1967 article[3] propose that, through the process of dilution and succession, the active substance acts as a template, communicating a field effect to the solvent through the formation of polymer chains (giant molecular aggregates) in the solvent. The three-dimensional structure of such polymers would be specific to each individual solute. Once the structural informational content of the solute has been transmitted to the solvent through the formation of polymer chains, the solute need no longer be present for the solvent to communicate that information to the human organism. How this quantum leap occurs remains unexplained; thus the riddle and ridicule of homeopathy.

In a 1977 article, Matthew Hubbard pointed out that when Avogadro formulated his law, matter was not believed to be divisible beyond the level of the atom. Now, of course, we have identified subatomic particles, and one comtemporary model defines atoms as ordered waves of energy. Thus, when we study the phenomena associated with apparently material substances, we are no longer restricted to the realm of matter; matter and energy, according to the first law of thermodynamics, are interchangeable and are constantly being transformed from one form to the other. As electrons jump from one orbit to another around the nucleus of the atom, radiation is released, which can be measured on a spectroscope. Each chemical element has its own spectroscopic "fingerprint," which is produced by this characteristic pattern of radiation. Hubbard proposes that the energy released from such molecules of matter must permeate an entire solution; thus, even if there is not a single atom of the original substance present in a highly diluted solution, the energy

3. G. P. Barnard and J. H. Stephenson, "Microdose Paradox: A New Biophysical Concept," *Journal of the American Institute of Homeopathy* (September-October 1967), vol. 60, pp. 277–86.

associated with this subatomic activity should be present in the solvent.[4]

The above two tentative approaches to the explanation of the activity of high potencies have some implications that can be tested in the laboratory. If there is a patterning of energy within the ultramolecular dilutions, these potencies should have physical and biological properties that distinguish them from samples of the solvent alone. In a series of experiments in the 1950s, A. Gay and J. Boiron demonstrated measurable differences between the capacitances (dielectric constants) of distilled water and of sodium chloride dissolved in distilled water and carried through stages of dilution up to 10^{-60}.[5]

The high potencies similarly have been shown to have effects in the biological sphere. In 1931, Paterson and Boyd showed that the Schick test, conventionally used to determine the presence or absence of immunity to diphtheria, can be altered through the administration of high potencies of either alum precipitated toxoid (APT)—used by allopaths in material doses to induce immunity—or of *Diphtherinum*, a nosode prepared from a diphtheritic membrane. Of the subjects who originally showed absence of immunity (Schick positive), a significant number showed immunity (Schick negative) after administration of one of the potentized substances.

During the 1930s, W. Persson demonstrated that the rate of fermentation of starch by the enzyme ptyalin could be influenced by high potencies of mercuric chloride, and that lysis of fibrin by the enzymes pepsin and trypsin could be influenced by high potencies of a number of different substances. In 1954, W. Boyd, after fifteen years of retesting Persson's findings, reported that the presence of dilutions of

4. Matthew Hubbard, "A 20th Century Critique of Avogadro's Law and Its Implications," *Journal of the American Institute of Homeopathy* (September 1977), pp. 433–36.

5. This study and the ones that follow are summarized in James Stephenson, M.D., "A Review of Investigations into the Action of Substances in Dilutions Greater than 1×10^{-24} (Microdilutions)," *Journal of the American Institute of Homeopathy* 48, no. 11 (November 1955): 327–35.

mercuric chloride up to 10^{-61} had a highly significant influence on the rate of hydrolysis of starch by the enzyme diastase, with the potentized mercuric chloride stimulating the process.

Similarly, other investigators have shown that high potencies can have an effect on the rate of growth of the mycelium of fungi, the rate of germination of barley and wheat germ, the transmission of nerve impulses in the human being, the physiological processes in animal organs, and the inheritance of genetically determined tumors in the fruit fly.

These studies, all cited by Stephenson, strongly suggest that the high potencies are capable of influencing physical and biological phenomena under controlled experimental conditions in the laboratory. Stephenson evaluated the methodology of these studies and concluded that they were well controlled. In order for such findings to gain credence among orthodox physicians and scientists, they would need to be duplicated many times under impeccably controlled conditions, and preferably by scientists who are not strongly associated with the homeopathic camp. This is not to imply that the results cited above are spurious, but rather it indicates the degree of resistance to homeopathy.

Homeopaths have tended to let the claims for Hahnemann's doctrine rest on the evidence of its success in clinical practice. Obviously some elements of the homeopathic doctrine are not susceptible to demonstration in the laboratory at the present stage of our scientific knowledge, but where such demonstration is possible, perhaps further laboratory studies would help to eliminate some of the hostility toward homeopathy.

COMPARATIVE CLINICAL STUDIES

An important factor in the spread and acceptance of homeopathy was its demonstrated clinical success in nineteenth-century epidemics. Such anecdotal evidence is hard to evaluate, for much of the success may have been due to the absense of positive harm (for example, the drugging, purging, or bleeding common in allopathic practice at the time) rather than to the efficacy of the remedies themselves.

With the relatively limited practice of homeopathy in the United States today, and with no homeopathic institutions in which clinical data can be collected, it is difficult to make comparisons between the clinical success of homeopathy and allopathy in this country. In England, where homeopathy has remained a strong force, such statistics are more readily available, and we shall mention two comparative studies.

Dr. Margery Blackie relates the story of a severe cholera epidemic in London in 1854, during which the facilities of the London Homeopathic Hospital were turned over completely to the treatment of cholera victims. Although the treatment of these patients was reportedly spectacularly successful, the Medical Council failed to report the results of the Homeopathic Hospital's treatment in their Blue Book of statistics. When the matter was brought up in Parliament, a separate Blue Book was issued to report the figures: as compared with a death rate in other hospitals of 51.8 percent, the London Homeopathic Hospital's death rate was only 16.4 percent in all true cholera cases.[6]

More recently, a survey was carried out in English factories and offices, comparing the results of allopathic and homeopathic treatment of influenza between 1968 and 1970.[7] The purpose of the survey was to determine the effectiveness of the homeopathic nosode *Influenzinum*, prepared from the influenza virus current at the time. Patients of allopathic physicians did not receive the homeopathic nosode, and 19.7 percent of them contracted the flu; among the homeopathically immunized patients, only 6.5 percent came down with the disease. Furthermore, the number of working days lost by allopathic patients was nearly eight and a half times greater than those lost by homeopathic patients, which seems to indicate that homeopathic patients who did become sick recovered considerably more rapidly than did the allopathic patients, thanks to the partial immunity conferred on them by the nosode.

6. Margery G. Blackie, *The Patient, Not the Cure* (London: Macdonald and Jane's, 1976), pp. 109–110.

7. D. H. Livingston et al., *Homeopathy* (November 1970), quoted in G. Ruthven Mitchell, *Homeopathy* (London: W. H. Allen, 1975), pp. 124–125.

It is hoped that, particularly in such countries as England where comparative studies can be made with relatively little difficulty, more statistical analyses will be done in the years to come.

USE OF THE COMPUTER IN REPERTORIZING

According to homeopathic theory, once the case is properly taken, the homeopath will be able to find the proper remedy for the patient's total symptom picture through a painstaking symptom-by-symptom analysis of the case, using the repertory to find all remedies corresponding to each symptom and its modalities. Theoretically, this search through the repertory could be conducted by a properly programmed computer.

Dr. Bhaghat Singh, who practices in New York, has devised such a program, and it is being used by a number of homeopathic physicians across the United States. The process starts with a case-taking form, which the patient fills out in the doctor's office. The first four pages of the form outline the patient's present illness, his past medical history, including any drugs he has taken, his family medical history, and the state of the health of his children. These routine items appear in virtually any medical history, and the doctor orders his thinking through this history, forming a picture of the patient's health. In the succeeding pages of the form, there is a checklist of some 980 symptoms from Kent's *Repertory*, and the patient indicates whether each symptom is currently present, whether he has ever had the symptom in the past, or whether he has never had the symptom. The information from this inventory is then fed into the computer, which repertorizes the symptoms in the classical way, adding up the probabilities and coming up with the three most likely remedies.

The doctor's judgment must still be brought to bear in evaluating the likelihood that any of the remedies suggested is the correct one. It is an axiom of computer science that the output of a program is only as good as the information put into it. Thus, a possible source of error could be that the form itself suggests symptoms to the patient. Moreover, without the skillful eliciting of each symptom by the physician, the patient might conceal certain symptoms and exaggerate others, and important modalities might be ignored. Although homeopaths tend to understate the aspect of "art" in homeopathic prescribing, there are obviously many steps in the process of taking and studying a case where the skill and judgment of the physician play a major role. Intuition is a strong force in any healing ritual.

In Kent's *Repertory*, symptoms are weighted according to grade, or the degree to which they are marked in the provings. Similarly, the patient's symptoms are weighted in the taking of the case. Dr. Singh has developed a new program that reflects the grades assigned to the remedies in the *Repertory*. It also indicates the frequency of each remedy— the number of times it came up in the repertorization, regardless of its weight under each individual rubric. This can be helpful, for homeopaths say that a remedy that runs through all symptoms might be more similar to the patient's total picture than a remedy that is strongly marked under only some of the rubrics, for which the patient's symptoms are also strongly marked. The new program also comes up with five suggested remedies instead of three.

Of course, the computer is nothing more than a calculating machine, but, if clinical experience indicates that it can be a helpful tool in homeopathic prescribing, it could save the physician considerable time which, ideally, could be devoted to taking the case in such a way that the input supplied to the computer would be of the highest, most reliable quality.

THE SCIENTIFIC STATUS OF HOMEOPATHY

Homeopathy, as much as allopathy, will make use of modern diagnostic tools and therapeutic procedures when they are judged to be of benefit to the patient.

Homeopathic thinking, based on the inductive method, begins with observation of the "real world" and proceeds to make hypotheses on the basis of such observation; it then tests its hypotheses against actual experience. Such methodology is certainly scientific when consistently carried out.

In a narrower sense, "scientific" refers to a theory or an idea that is potentially *disprovable*. According to this analysis, if an idea is not potentially disprovable, it is meaningless. Does homeopathy meet this definition?

What kind of evidence would theoretically invalidate the homeopathic doctrine? Obviously, any experience that showed that like did *not* cure like could be taken as evidence that the Law of Similars was incorrect. In reality, however, when a prescription based on the Law of Similars fails to effect a cure, homeopathic advocates blame the prescriber, not the homeopathic doctrine. Homeopaths insist that correct prescribing is an extremely difficult task and that failures in practice should not be taken as evidence against the correctness of the homeopathic doctrine.

It would appear that the "artistic" element of homeopathy is considerably greater than homeopathic theorists concede, for if the doctrine is so difficult to apply, then it must take an exceptionally insightful and gifted prescriber to achieve clinical success with any consistency.

In contrast to their reluctance to admit the evidence of failures in clinical trials, homeopaths have openly advocated the laboratory investigation of the activity of the high potencies. A great deal of work remains to be done, although preliminary findings seem to indicate that some potentized homeopathic remedies do exhibit properties that suggest they might be active within the human organism. Further experimentation with the high potencies, as well as modern reprovings of the remedies under well-designed double-blind conditions, would go a long way toward establishing that homeopathy is capable of standing up under the scrutiny of contemporary scientific evaluation.

PART II

SOME TOOLS FOR THE PRACTICE OF HOMEOPATHY

6

HOMEOPATHIC
REMEDIES

A SURVEY OF THE REMEDIES

The homeopathic materia medica comprises some two thousand different substances derived from the animal, vegetable, and mineral kingdoms, as well as some remedies classed as "imponderabilia," such as X ray, which is a potentization of alcohol that has been exposed to X rays. Of course, there are some shadings between the three great kingdoms: for example, Calcarea carbonica, or calcium carbonate, although it is a mineral salt, is derived for homeopathic use from oyster shell, rather than from mineral deposits.

Among the mineral substances used are mineral elements and salts that have been demonstrated to play an important role in the functioning of the living organism. Some of the most frequently used homeopathic remedies, including sulfur, *natrum muriaticum* (sodium chloride, or table salt), cuprum (copper), and Silicea (silica), occur in the human either as trace elements or as important building blocks of body tissues. Other minerals, such as arsenic, mercury, and phosphorus, are extremely toxic to the human organism, yet, when they are prepared as homeopathic potencies, their toxicity is removed and they have applications in a broad range of complaints.

Some of the mineral remedies, such as silica, are generally considered medicinally inert outside the practice of homeopathy; others, such as common table salt, are recognized as playing a role in the functioning of the organism, but are believed to have limited use as drugs. However, through the process of potentization, hitherto unsuspected properties are brought out in such substances, and they can then be used as medicines.

The vegetable remedies include plants that have had long use as medicines, as well as those that have long been known to produce toxic effects. *Belladonna, chamomilla,* and *ipecacuanha,* for example, have been valued for centuries for their medicinal properties. Interestingly, *Belladonna* has also been used as a poison, as have nux vomica (strychnine), aconite, and others. The vegetable remedies also include plants whose medicinal value was virtually unknown before they were used by homeopaths: *Lycopodium* is an example. Generally, food plants are not employed as homeopathic remedies, since as foods they should not have drug effects, but a few foods, such as the onion, have obvious effects and are frequently employed. Since some people have idiosyncrasies to certain kinds of foods, the materia medica also includes some incompletely proved foods, such as celery, grapefruit, tomato, and cane sugar.[1]

The animal-derived remedies are particularly interesting. They include the venoms of a number of animals, including the bee, various poisonous snakes, and the tarantula, all of which when potentized have a wide range of applications. Sepia, or the ink of the cuttlefish, is an example of a commonly employed animal remedy that was considered inert before it was introduced by Hahnemann.

Another group of remedies, known as the *nosodes,* are derived from disease material: pus, bacteria, etc. The nosodes are usually identified by the suffix *-inum.* Before vaccination was introduced into allopathy, homeopaths had already been potentizing some disease products, such as lyssin, the saliva of the rabid dog, to treat victims of the respective diseases. Employment of a substance that is identical with the disease, rather than a substance that is similar, is known as *isopathy.* Isopathy enjoyed considerable popularity in the United States

1. Hering observed that many chronic diseases of women and children are the results of using too much sugar; this observation on the drug effects of sugar anticipates the recent concern about the ill effects of overconsumption of this substance.

during the time when the idea of vaccination became widespread, but today American homeopaths prefer to prescribe on the totality of the patient's symptoms rather than on the basis of a suspected disease-producing organism. There are incomplete provings for many of the nosodes, and homeopaths might be able to prescribe them more widely if the symptom pictures calling for them were more complete. In other countries, particularly in Germany and England, nosodes are wisely used isopathically by homeopaths, both to treat acute diseases and as a preventative in epidemics. For example, potencies of *influenzinum*, or influenza virus, may be prepared to confer immunity on patients in a flu epidemic.

While routine prescribing of nosodes along isopathic lines is generally not considered good homeopathic practice in this country, the strictest interpreters of Hahnemann's doctrine agree that the nosodes can be of great value in the treatment of chronic diseases. They are used not only to break up the lingering effects of a disease, such as flu or tuberculosis, but also to reach deep into the constitutional pattern of a patient and clear a chronic miasm that was implanted long in the past through exposure to a disease, through vaccination, or through inheritance. Thus, for example, *medorrhinum* (from gonorrhea), *psorinum* (from scabies), *syphilinum* (from syphilis), and *tuberculinum* (from tuberculosis) are reported to be helpful in many cases when there is a history of infection, either in the individual patient or in his parents. Often, when the carefully selected homeopathic remedy fails to act, homeopaths report that a dose of the appropriate nosode, determined from the patient's history, will either clear up the case by itself or cause the patient to respond subsequently to the indicated remedy. Nosodes are similarly credited with breaking up the periodicity of chronic diseases; whereas each individual flare-up of a chronic condition may respond to the proper remedy, it may take a nosode to prevent the pattern of recurrence.

Remedies that have produced a wide range of symptoms in provers, and therefore have a broad range of application in the treatment of illness, are known as *polychrests*. The term, meaning "many uses," was coined by Hahnemann from the Greek, and was first used in his 1817 article on nux vomica in volume 2 of the *Materia Medica Pura.* Because the polychrests in their provings demonstrate an ability to affect every part of the organism, they are particularly adapted to constitutional prescribing, in which the homeopath is matching the total constitutional picture of the patient—every aspect of his physical, emotional, and mental state—to a drug that similarly manifests activity in every sphere of the healthy human organism.

In the following pages, some of the most widely used homeopathic remedies are discussed in some detail. The sources of the remedies are identified, and even among the limited number of medicines included, you will note a great diversity. In order to place the remedies in historical, social, and scientific perspective, there is a brief discussion of the use of each substance in allopathic medicine, in folk medicine, and in other applications, as well as what is known about its chemical action in the human body.

The subsequent paragraphs under each remedy summarize the symptom image as described in leading works on the homeopathic materia medica. The symptoms are arranged in a specific order. The first paragraph describes the general symptoms produced by the drug, including observations on the constitutional type of the patient most likely to respond to the remedy. Important modalities are included in a discussion of the generals. The next paragraph details the mental picture of the remedy. The final paragraph describes the particulars in the following order: head, eyes, ears, nose, mouth, throat, stomach, abdomen, stool, urine, male, female, respiratory, back, extremities, skin, fever. Finally, some of the prominent modalities are given; that is, what generally makes the symptoms better and what makes them worse. In some cases, important relationships with other remedies are also mentioned. Only a relatively few prominent symptoms can be included in the treatments herein; in a complete materia medica, many of the remedies have thousands of symptoms.

ACONITUM NAPELLUS (Monkshood, Wolfsbane)
(ăk-o-nī′tŭm nā-pel′lŭs)

Identification: *Aconitum napellus*, or, more commonly, Aconite, is a perennial herb of the family Ranunculaceae, common in wet, hilly areas. It grows from two to six feet in height and has bluish violet hooded flowers. The tincture is prepared from the whole plant and root, gathered at the beginning of flowering.

Drug Action: The active principle in Aconite is the alkaloid aconitine, a deadly poison; the root possesses nine times the strength of the leaf. It first stimulates, then depresses the sensory nerve endings, especially those of sensation; it stimulates the medullary inhibitory heart center, producing slowed pulse. It also has a direct depressive effect on the respiratory center, sometimes producing death through inhibition of breathing before the heart fails.

History: Mentioned in the writings of the classical Greek writers, aconite was used as a poison in ancient times and during the Middle Ages. It was introduced into medicine by Anton von Stoerck, who in 1762 reported using aconite internally for various conditions and concluded that it worked by promoting evacuations. In the latter eighteenth century, other physicians took up its use, but there developed a feeling that it was too dangerous for internal use, although it was still used topically.

Hahnemann published his provings of Aconite in 1805, and it rapidly became one of the most widely used remedies in homeopathy, particularly in diseases characterized by fever and inflammation. It became the homeopathic substitute for bloodletting, hence was nicknamed the "homeopathic lancet." Orthodox medicine began using Aconite once again after its introduction into homeopathy, and among allopaths as well it acquired a reputation for being a safer and more reliable treatment than bloodletting, although bleeding still had its staunch defenders. Both bleeding and Aconite continued to be used in allopathic medicine up to World War I.

Symptoms and Uses: Aconite is a fast-acting medicine. Its effects are short in duration, and it must be repeated frequently in acute conditions. Its principal sphere of use is in complaints that come on suddenly and with great intensity. The Aconite patient is generally a vigorous, plethoric individual whose complaints are brought on shortly after exposure to cold, dry air. It also is used for complaints that come on suddenly from the intense heat of summer. In its provings, Aconite is shown to produce functional disturbances, but not to continue its action into tissue change; it is therefore suited to the beginning of an acute disease, but when body tissues begin to be affected by a disease, a change of remedy is called for. Aconite has traditionally been considered the remedy of choice at the very first signs of a cold, although patients in the twentieth century do not seem as susceptible to this remedy as were patients in earlier times. Aconite is associated with inflammatory conditions throughout the body, with intensity of sensation. The pains are stinging, burning, cutting, stabbing; the patient screams with pain. Aconite conditions are associated with dryness and redness. The aconite patient is very thirsty, craving large quantities of cold water.

The mental symptoms are of prime importance. There is intense anxiety, restlessness, nervous irritation, and excitement. Fear shows on the face. Ailments are accompanied by anxiety. The symptoms are so intense and come on so suddenly that the patient fears he will die, even predicting the hour of his death.

The Aconite headache comes on with great violence. Tearing, burning, congestive headache with anxiety, hot red face, anxious expression. Vertigo. Neuralgic pains in the face from exposure to dry cold. Intense sensitivity of hearing; noise or music are intolerable. Runny nose with sneezing, coming on in the night after exposure to cold during the day; mucous membranes of nose are dry. Sore throat, dry, red, burning, smarting. Acute inflammation of the stomach; burning, tearing pains. The patient desires large quantities of cold water. Catarrhal inflammations of all the abdominal organs. Sudden inflammation of the liver. Vomiting bright red blood. Bowel complaints in children, from intense summer heat. Inflammatory conditions of kidneys and bladder. Urine hot, dark, red, scanty. Retention of urine from shock; retention of urine in the newborn from the shock of delivery. Symptoms in women after difficult parturition, attended with fear and restlessness. Inflammatory conditions in the chest. Shortness of breath associated with cardiac excitement, in plethoric individuals after exposure to cold, after shock. Dry cough; whole chest feels dry. Sudden attacks of pain in heart with hard, full pulse. Acute rheumatic conditions of the joints after sudden exposure to cold. Numbness and tingling along the nerves from exposure to cold. Sensation of insects crawling on spine. The skin is red, hot, swollen, dry. Formication and numbness. Fever with dry heat, red face; cold stage with thirst, restlessness.

Modalities: Worse: warm room; evening and night; lying on affected side; music; tobacco smoke; dry, cold winds. Better: open air, after sweating, rest.

Relationships: Sulfur often completes aconite cases. *Arnica* and *Belladonna* also follow Aconite well.

APIS MELLIFICA (Honeybee)
(ā′pĭs mĕl-lĭf′ĭ-ka)

Identification: *Apis* is prepared from live bees of the genus *Apis*, the common hive bee. The population of the hive consists of one queen, several hundred male drones, and ten thousand or so undeveloped female worker bees. Only the queen and the worker bees have the poison apparatus, or stinger. The live bees are placed in a bottle; the bottle is shaken to irritate them, and alcohol is added. After ten days, with the bottle shaken twice daily, the tincture is poured off. Although only the contents of the poison sacs are desired for their medicinal value, the solution will also contain other animal fluids, honey, and pollen. Serial dilutions are prepared from the tincture.

History: There was a popular belief in folk medicine that beestings cured rheumatism. *Apis* was proved by a homeopath in 1835, and extensive provings were published by Hering in 1857. In the late nineteenth century, some allopaths, taking their cue from the homeopathic uses of bee venom, reported success in treating rheumatism and rheumatoid arthritis, and since that time, *Apis* has been popular periodically in allopathic practice. Honeybee antigen is an ingredient in a stinging insect antigen used by allopaths today to desensitize patients to stinging insect reactions. It is available in serial dilutions for this purpose and is injected subcutaneously. A substance in bee venom, Peptide 401, has recently been shown by allopathic researchers to be one hundred times as effective as cortisone in treating rheumatism in animals.

Symptoms and Uses: The symptom picture of *Apis* resembles the effects of a beesting: edéma, redness, and sharp, stinging pains. *Apis* acts on cellular tissues, specifically of outer parts— the skin, the mucous membranes, and the tissues that cover internal organs—producing edema, inflammation, stinging, and burning. *Apis* is used to treat the bad effects of suppressed acute eruptions, as in measles. Complaints calling for *Apis* come on rapidly and are violent in intensity. Heat aggravates all symptoms. The affected parts are extremely sensitive to touch. In many complaints there is a sensation of tightness or constriction. Many symptoms begin on the right and spread to the left. The action of *Apis* may be relatively slow.

The mental symptoms include apathy, drowsiness, sadness, tearfulness without cause, suspiciousness, jealousy, irritability. There is a disturbance of coordination, awkwardness; the patient drops things readily. With the congestion of the brain there is a characteristic shriek. The patient screams and starts suddenly from sleep.

Congestion of the brain. Heat, throbbing, distensive pains in the head, worse from heat, worse from motion, better from pressure. An erysipelatous, red, swollen rash appears on the face, with stinging, burning pains; beginning on the right, spreading to the left. The eyes have swollen, edematous red lids, everted, inflamed, burning, stinging, with hot tears. The throat shows swelling in all its parts, with burning, stinging pains, better from cold, worse from heat. Tonsillitis with water-bag appearance of the uvula. Aversion to all warm substances. The *Apis* patient is thirstless. Sensation of soreness and tightness throughout the abdomen; abdomen is edamatous. Bruised feeling of the intestines. The urine is hot and bloody. Urging to urinate as soon as a few drops collect in the bladder. Inflammation of the kidneys, ureters, bladder, urethra. Burning and soreness on urination. There is edematous swelling of the feet and limbs, with pitting on pressure; burning, stinging, and numbness in the limbs. Rheumatic pain in back and limbs. Awkwardness of the fingers, toes, and limbs. The skin shows a thick, rough rash, often rosy in color, worse from heat. The skin is extremely sensitive to touch. *Apis* is often useful in beestings and insect bites. In fever, the patient is worse from heat, even during a chill; kicks off the covers while shivering.

Modalities: Worse: heat, touch, pressure, late in afternoon, right side, closed room. Better: open air, cold applications, uncovering.

Relationships: *Natrum muriaticum* is the chronic counterpart of *Apis*; also *Baryta carbonica* if the lymphatics are involved.

ARNICA MONTANA (Mountain Arnica, Leopard's-bane, Mountain Tobacco, Wolfsbane)
(är′nĭ-ka mŏn-tā′na)

Identification: *Arnica montana* is a perennial herb of the family Compositae that grows in the moist, cool upland meadows or mountains of Europe; it is also found sparsely in the northwestern United States. It stands ten to twelve inches high and has a dull green involucre with purplish hairy points and a tubular corolla with five spreading teeth. The disc flowers are yellow and numerous. The whole fresh plant, including the root, is commonly used to make the tincture; more recently, after the eggs of a parasitical fly were discovered on the flowers, the root alone has also been used.

History and Drug Action: Experimental studies in animals or in humans have reinforced folk usage of *Arnica* flowers as emollients, to promote wound healing, and to reduce inflammation of nasal passages. Internally, herbal preparations have been used for high blood pressure and for various heart disorders. *Arnica* was a popular household remedy in the early nineteenth century in Europe, used topically for cuts, bruises, and sprains. Hahnemann published provings of *Arnica* in 1805, and it soon became a widely used homeopathic remedy, not only for external application, but also given internally in potencies. There was considerable resistance among allopaths to the use of *Arnica* because it had been popularized by homeopathy. Although some allopaths claimed it was inert, others used it in the nineteenth century both in the traditional manner and for the purposes introduced by homeopathy.

Symptoms and Uses: *Arnica* is an important remedy in injuries, sprains, bruises, and shock, and when the symptoms agree, it is the first remedy given after such trauma. Used topically as a tincture, oil, or ointment, it may be applied to injured parts, but only if the skin is unbroken. Given internally in potencies, it is credited with saving lives and speeding recovery after trauma. There is a characteristic bruised, sore feeling throughout the body, as if the patient has been beaten; athletes rub down with *Arnica* to counteract the effects of muscular overexertion. The patient is restless, turning and moving because he is so sore he can only lie or sit in one position for a short time. Bed feels too hard. *Arnica* is reported to control hemorrhages and promote reabsorption of blood. Offensive discharges. The body is cold, the head hot. *Arnica* is valued as a remedy for the aftereffects of injuries, even when remote in time.

The mental state of the *Arnica* patient is one of prostration and stupor. The patient wants to be let alone; does not want to be talked to and does not want to be touched. He can be roused from his stupor to answer a question, then he sinks back. Sends the doctor away, even when seriously ill. Shock state. Stupor from concussion. Horrors in the night; awakens, grasping at his heart; cardiac distress in the night, even in the absence of heart disease. Nightmares. Sleepless and restless when overtired.

Head hot, with cold body. Face is apoplectic, red. Bruised, sore feeling in eyes after close work. Dry mouth; the patient is thirsty. Fetid breath. Bitter taste; taste of bad eggs. Soreness of gums after tooth extraction. Aversion to meat and milk. Inflammatory conditions of abdomen, liver, intestines. Abdomen sore; cannot be touched. Black vomit; vomiting blood. Offensive stool and flatus. Black stools. Urine retention from overexertion. Pregnant women have feeling of soreness throughout body; sensitive to motion of fetus. Bruised feeling of pelvic organs after labor. Helps prevent complications following childbirth. In the cardiovascular system there is venous stasis, with bruising and hemorrhage. Angina pectoris; stitches in heart. Pulse feeble, irregular. Cardiac dropsy, shortness of breath. The extremities show rheumatic lameness; joints are swollen and sore. Traumatic affections of muscles. Gout. Does not want the extremities touched. Pain in back and limbs, as if bruised or beaten. Sprained, dislocated feeling. Soreness after overexertion. Black-and-blue marks on skin. Fever resembling the low sort of typhoid fever.

Modalities: Worse: touch, motion, rest, wine, damp cold. Better: lying down, or with head low.

Relationships: Follows aconite well in injuries.

ARSENICUM ALBUM (Arsenic Trioxide (As_2O_3), White Oxide of Arsenic, Arsenious Acid, Arsenic)
(är-sĕn'ĭ-kŭm ăl'bŭm)

Identification: Arsenic trioxide when freshly prepared consists of large, vitreous amorphous masses that gradually become opaque, crystalline, and porcelainlike. It is barely soluble in alcohol and soluble in water and alkalies. Arsenic is found in nature and extracted from its ore. The potencies are prepared either by trituration or as a tincture containing arsenic in water and alcohol, with a strength of 1/100.

Drug Action: Arsenic is a deadly poison in crude form. It is believed that trivalent arsenical compounds react with sulfhydryl groups in the cells, inhibiting sulfhydryl enzymes essential to cellular metabolism. When applied topically, arsenic poisons the skin tissue, causing corrosion and sloughing. In large doses it damages the blood vessels, interferes with the cellular composition of blood, and ultimately leads to tissue and organ damage throughout the body.

History: Arsenic was an ancient therapeutic agent used by the Greeks and Romans. It was popular as a poisoning agent up to the first quarter of the twentieth century. Hahnemann introduced arsenic into homeopathy and documented the symptoms in *Chronic Diseases* (1828). Organic compounds of arsenic were used early in allopathic chemotherapy, and they were used in many "quack" remedies such as "cancer pastes" that were supposed to destroy accessible tumors. Animal fanciers and breeders have used arsenic preparations to improve the skin and fur of animals. Arsenic compounds have been used as a "tonic" to enhance endurance, as in mountain climbing, and allopaths previously treated pernicious anemia with arsenicals. The only present allopathic use of arsenical compounds is in the treatment of tropical parasitic diseases. Arsenic is still used in pesticides and is a cause of accidental poisoning in humans.

Symptoms and Uses: *Arsenicum album* is one of the most frequently used polychrests, since it is capable of affecting every part of the body. There is great prostration; exhaustion after the slightest exertion. The body is pale, cold, clammy, and the patient has a cadaveric appearance. The Arsenic patient is very chilly, and symptoms are generally better from warmth, except for the head symptoms, which are better from cold (external head is better from warmth). Sudden rapid inflammatory conditions with a tendency to gangrene. Secretions and excretions are acrid, excoriating the parts they contact. Burning sensation through all the complaints. Putrid odor of discharges, like decomposing flesh. Frequent thirst for small quantities, although the patient may be thirstless. Most symptoms are worse after midnight, especially between 1:00 and 2:00 A.M. Periodic complaints; the more chronic the problem, the longer the interval. Alternation of states as in many antipsoric remedies; head symptoms alternating with physical symptoms.

The mental symptoms are characterized by anxiety. There is great anxiety with restlessness; the patient constantly moves from one place to a another. Anxiety about sickness; fear of death; mind always occupied with anxious thoughts about important or unimportant details. The anxiety is reflected in a pronounced fastidiousness; patient is very sensitive to disorder and confusion; every picture on the wall of the sickroom must hang straight. The Arsenic patient is known as the "gold-headed cane patient" because of his fastidiousness and attention to dress. Patient can be domineering, critical, intolerant because of his anxious obsession with detail. Suicidal tendencies. Dreads solitude; wants company. Depression, sadness, despair. As the *Arsenicum* state progresses, the anxiety and restlessness give way to great weakness, prostration. Oversensitivity of all senses, especially smell and touch.

Periodical headaches, often with nausea and vomiting; better from cold. Scalp is so sensitive to touch that the hair cannot be combed. Face waxy and pale; edema of face and head; cadaveric appearance. Catarrhal conditions of the eyes with excoriating, burning discharges. Always taking cold in the nose; sneezes with every change of weather; worse in cold damp weather. Excoriating discharge from the nose. Later stages of colds, with red nose and eyes, sneezing, profuse discharges; patient is chilly. Colds begin in the nose, moving into the throat with hoarseness, dry, rasping cough. Redness and shriveling of the mucous membranes. Gastritis, vomiting everything taken. Dry mouth. Burning pains throughout the digestive tract. Distention of abdomen; tympanitic, as in peritonitis. Stomach sensitive to touch. External heat and warm drinks relieve symptoms of stomach and abdomen. Intestinal colic from food poisoning. Stool has cadaveric odor like putrid flesh. Diarrhea, dysentery. Stools burn, excoriate the parts they pass over, causing redness and burning. Diarrhea alternating with constipation. Hot, dry hemorrhoids with burning sensation. Burning eruptions, spreading ulcers on genitals. In the male, swollen penis, swollen scrotum. In the female, burning pains in the genitals; excoriating leukorrhea, itching and burning. Burning in chest; catarrhal conditions spreading down into the chest with dry, hacking cough; later, excoriating expectoration. Asthma of nervous character. Cardiac weakness; palpitation from least exertion; shortness of breath. *Arsenicum* corresponds to many serious, often incurable complaints of the heart. Anemia. Shriveling of skin; dry, rough, scaly skin eruptions; ulcers with offensive discharge; gangrenous inflammations. Intermittent fevers.

Modalities: Worse: after midnight (1:00 to 2:00 A.M., 1:00 to 2:00 P.M.), cold, cold drinks or food, right side. Better: heat, head elevated, warm drinks.

AURUM METALLICUM (Metallic Gold)
(au′rŭm mĕ-tăl′lĭ-kŭm)

Identification: Metallic gold is extremely unreactive chemically; it is insoluble in water and in sulfuric and nitric acids; it is soluble in aqua regia (a combination of nitric and hydrochloric acids). It occurs in its pure form in nature. The homeopathic gold, a fine brown powder, is obtained as a precipitate from the chloride. The lower potencies are prepared by trituration, since gold is not soluble in water or alcohol.

History: In 1890 Robert Koch reported that the tubercle bacillus was adversely affected by low concentrations of gold salts. After that time gold in the form of aurous salts was used in tuberculosis and syphilis in allopathic practice. More recently, allopaths have used gold salt injections on an experimental basis in treating arthritis and nondisseminated lupus erythematosus. In the past, gold compounds were also used in allopathy to treat uveitis, but newer drugs have replaced gold for this purpose. In the allopathic applications mentioned above, gold has been noted to have toxic effects, including disturbances of the skin and mucous membranes, blood disorders, and other organic problems. Hahnemann in his *Chronic Diseases* (1828) reports on the symptoms from provings of *Aurum*.

In alchemy, gold is equated with the essence of the sun, the arcanum of warmth and life in the heart. Also, in its "black sun" form, it represents the opposite—decay, putrefaction, and death. Symbolically, gold is equated with the life force, the ego, the blood.

Symptoms and Uses: Considered medicinally inert in its pure state, gold in its potentized form finds applications in homeopathy in disturbances of the mind and the body tissues in general. Prominent in the symptom picture of *Aurum* are disorders resembling the symptoms of secondary syphilis and mercury poisoning, affecting the bones, glands, and blood; gouty tendency of joints; cardiac disturbances.

The mental symptoms of *Aurum* are striking. The affections are deranged; the patient has no love of life, is hopeless, melancholy, depressed, has no enjoyment. Self-reproachful; imagines he has neglected his duty; concerned about his salvation. The future looks dark. There are marked suicidal tendencies; seeks out ways to commit suicide. Loathing of life. Sits and broods, saying nothing. Very irritable; when disturbed, aroused to great anger, violence. Restless, always in a hurry. Despair from severe pain.

Violent, congestive head pain, worse at night. Exostoses as in syphilis. The skull bones are painful and sensitive to touch. Catarrhal disturbances of the eyes; inflammation of conjunctivas, choroid, iris, retina. Extreme photophobia. Caries of the bones of the ear. Oversensitive to noise, but music relieves. Offensive, fetid discharge from nose. Necrosis of bones of nose, mastoid bones. Loss of smell. The glands everywhere are involved, with inflammation, hardness, enlargement. Liver inflamed, hard, enlarged. Appetite and thirst increased, with qualmishness. Inguinal glands swollen and suppurative. Pain and swelling of testicles, with hardness. Uterus enlarged and prolapsed. Asthma; shortness of breath of cardiac origin, shortness of breath at night. Kent notes that when the affections are deranged in mental disease, we find disease in the heart; whereas when the intellect is disturbed, it is the lungs that are affected. In *Aurum*, then, there are prominent heart symptoms. Enlargement of the heart; palpitation. Pulse rapid, feeble, irregular. Veins enlarged, inflamed, friable. Arteriosclerosis, high blood pressure. In the extremities there are symptoms of syphilitic and mercurial character; affections of the cartilage and bone, inflammation of the periosteum. Destruction of bones as in secondary syphilis. Rheumatic swelling of the joints. Violent, tearing pains in the limbs, worse at night. Edema of the extremities, with pitting on pressure. In the characteristic pattern of rheumatic affections, pains wander from joint to joint, finally settling in the heart.

Modalities: Worse: cold air, from sunset to sunrise, mental exertion, winter. Better: warm air, morning, summer.

BELLADONNA (Deadly Nightshade, *Atropa belladonna*)
(bĕl-la-dŏn′na)

Identification: *Atropa belladonna* is a large, bushy perennial herb of the family Solanaceae. The stem is erect and branching; the flowers are single, five lobed and bell shaped, dull reddish to purplish, tinged with pale green below. The whole plant gives off a fetid odor when bruised and stains a dark purplish color. The tincture is prepared from the whole plant when the plant is beginning to flower.

Drug Action: *Belladonna*, along with several other plants of the Solanaceae family, contains the potent alkaloids atropine, hyoscyamine, and hyoscine (scopolamine) in all parts of the plant, with atropine being the principal alkaloid. Atropine is a central nervous system stimulant, with its principal sphere of action in the medulla and higher cortical centers. In small and moderate doses, the effect is one of central excitation; with large doses the stimulation is followed by depression, coma, medullary paralysis, and death.

History: *Atropa belladonna* derives its name from Atropos, the Fate who cuts the thread of life. The plant was formerly widely used as a poison. Italian women used it in drops to dilate the pupils of their eyes, and it was used as a wash to remove pimples. Either of these uses might account for the name *belladonna*, or "beautiful lady." The drug was in use in Hahnemann's time for a variety of conditions. Even before Hahnemann published his provings in 1805, he had been interested in the potential of *Belladonna* as a cure for scarlet fever, a commonly fatal children's disease, since the symptoms he had observed in accidental poisonings resembled those of the disease. Eventually Hahnemann popularized the use of *Belladonna* not only as a cure, but as a preventative, of scarlet fever. This use passed into allopathy and was common in orthodox practice up to the end of the nineteenth century.

The *Belladonna* alkaloids have many applications in contemporary allopathic practice. As eye drops, they are used to dilate the pupil and paralyze visual accommodation in eye examination and in treating eye diseases. Atropinelike drugs are used in a wide variety of clinical conditions: to inhibit the effects of parasympathetic nervous system activity; in anesthesia; in cold preparations to reduce respiratory secretions; for bronchodilation; after heart attacks; as an antidote in organophosphorous insecticide poisoning and in fast-acting mushroom poisoning.

Symptoms and Uses: *Belladonna* is a relatively short-acting remedy with a characteristic pattern to all its complaints: symptoms come on suddenly, stay for a while, reach a peak of intensity, and then subside suddenly. *Belladonna* may therefore be repeated frequently in acute diseases. Heat accompanies all inflammatory complaints; the patient feels very hot to the touch. There is a subjective sensation of burning of affected parts, as well as the objective heat of the patient. Throbbing is another prominent symptom; throbbing of the carotids; throbbing of affected parts. *Belladonna* is also full of spasms, especially of circular fibers around various organs, with clutching sensation; convulsions in infants and in children with high fever. Hot head and cold extremities. Many symptoms are predominantly right-sided.

The mental symptoms are marked by irritability of the nerve centers, with oversensitivity of all the senses; sensitive to light, noise, touch; patient cannot bear to have the bed touched for fear of its being jarred. Excitement, rage; striking, biting; children are very disobedient and quarrelsome; the patient does strange things. Starting in sleep or at the approach of others. Anxiety, fear. Acute mania; patient has to be restrained. Delirium in fever. Violent dreams, nightmares, restless sleep.

Vertigo, worse moving head. Sensitive scalp; cannot have hair bound up or combed. Congestive headaches, sensitive to motion, jarring, slightest noise, light draft; throbbing. Head symptoms worse lying down. Headaches brought on by exposure to cold air, even having hair cut. Headache worse on right side. Face flushed, red, hot, skin shiny. Violent face aches, worse right side. Twitchings of face. Eyes red, glaring; dilated pupils. Intense photophobia. Dryness of mucous membranes of mouth, nose, tongue, throat. Great liability to take cold; sensitivity to drafts. Sore throat, especially on the right, with constriction on swallowing, enlargement and inflammation of the glands about the neck. Averse to water. Clutching pains of gallstone colic. Inflammatory conditions of stomach and bowels, with pain, burning, distention, sensitive to jarring, slightest motion, slightest pressure. Dysentery. Hemorrhoids, painful, red, cannot be touched. Marked irritation of bladder and urinary tract. Spasmodic clutching at the neck of the bladder. Suppression of urine. Bearing down sensation in the female reproductive system; feeling as if organs would protrude, sensitive to touch. Hemorrhage after childbirth, with hot blood. Menstrual pains, like labor, from contraction of circular fibers. Pains in ovary, especially right. Respiratory complaints with dry, spasmodic cough from clutching sensation in larynx. Loss of voice. Chest painful, tight. Pneumonia, pleurisy, especially right. Neuralgic pains of the legs, better from motion, coming on at rest. Swollen joints, hot, red, burning. Convulsive movements of the limbs; cramping. Cold extremities. Skin dry, hot, burning. Inflamed parts first very red, then dusky, then mottled. Fine red glossy rash on almost any inflamed surface; smooth scarlet fever rash. Passive redness of skin; when scratched by the fingernail it leaves a white line.

Modalities: Worse: touch, jar, noise, draft, after 3:00 P.M., lying down. Better: semierect.

Relationships: *Calcarea* is complementary, especially in chronic and constitutional diseases.

BRYONIA ALBA (Wild Bryony, White Bryony, Wild Hops)
(brī-ō′ne-a al′ba)

Identification: *Bryonia alba* is a perennial climbing vine of the family Cucurbitaceae, growing wild in European vineyards and woods and cultivated in the United States. It has a long, branched spindle-shaped root with a disagreeable taste and odor that disappear on drying. The flowers are small and greenish yellow, the berries black and globular. The tincture is prepared from the fresh root before flowering.

Drug Action: *Bryonia* contains a glucoside, bryonin, and a resin called bryoresin. The activity of the plant is in its resin. It has produced serious, even fatal poisoning.

History: *Bryonia* was known to ancient doctors; it is mentioned by Dioscorides and was used in ancient times for dropsy. *Bryonia* had applications as a cathartic, a remedy for rheumatic conditions, a purgative, and for pleurisy, although it was not in great use by Hahnemann's time. Hahnemann introduced *Bryonia* into homeopathy through his proving in 1816; homeopaths began to use it in cholera, typhus, typhoid, and other conditions, including pneumonia and rheumatic problems, headaches and neuralgias. Eventually nineteenth-century allopathic physicians used *Bryonia* as a specific for the same conditions.

Symptoms and Uses: *Bryonia* is a polychrest with deep-seated, slow action. Acute complaints susceptible to *Bryonia* develop slowly, increasing to violent proportions. *Bryonia* is therefore suitable to continued fevers, rheumatic complaints of gradually increasing severity. It acts especially on the fibrous tissues, also the serous membranes, ligaments, and aponeuroses, and it congests the coatings of nerves. Extreme dryness of the mucous membranes. The *Bryonia* patient is of a venous, sluggish, plethoric constitution, with poor circulation. *Bryonia* illnesses are more likely to appear in warm, damp climates. The *Bryonia* patient goes through a long prodromal period, not feeling very well, languid; gradually the illness increases; pains flit about, finally becoming steady, continuous pain. Complaints are worse from the least motion of any sort. Many symptoms are worse from heat, but some are worse from cold. Many complaints are worse on the right side, or right-sided.

The mental state is characterized by irritability and dullness of mind. The patient doesn't want to answer questions or to talk. The mind is sluggish, going in severe cases into complete stupefaction and unconsciousness. Mental symptoms are better from cool fresh air, worse from the least motion or from being talked to. Low, passive form of delirium; patient wakes and wants to go home, doesn't know where he is. Talks of business in his delirium. Wants things that cannot be had; refuses things asked for when they are offered. Children dislike to be carried. Anxiety, uneasy feeling compels patient to move, which makes him worse. Anger worsens symptoms. Fear, anxiety, despair of recovery, despondency.

There are violent, congestive, bursting headaches; inflammation of the membranes of the brain and sometimes of the spinal cord. Headaches are worse from altercations, controversy. Dizziness. Headaches accompany every acute complaint, inflammatory and congestive complaints; worse from a warm room, motion, even moving the eyeballs; patient must keep perfectly still. The face is puffed, purplish, mottled, showing venous stasis. The countenance is dull, besotted, imbecilic. In congestive attacks, there is a peculiar chewing motion of the jaw; jaw wags back and forth. Eyes are sore on motion, on touch. Many complaints begin in the nose with sneezing and running nose and then move down into throat and larynx, developing into bronchitis, pneumonia, or pleurisy. Nosebleeds with congestion, coryza, instead of menstrual flow. Lips, tongue, and mouth dry. Great thirst for large quantities of water. Disordered stomach, with hiccup, belching, nausea, and vomiting; worse from eating. Abdomen sore to pressure. Inflammation of liver; sore and tender to pressure. Constipation; stools hard, dry, large. Diarrhea in hot weather. Colds with loss of voice, rawness in trachea; soreness in chest; dry racking cough; holds chest when coughing; pain mostly on right side. Right-sided pneumonia with rusty sputum. Panting breathing; rapid, short breaths because deep breathing increases pain. Pleurisy, with sharp, stitching pains, worse from motion. In the female, painful menstruation; suppressed menses, with vicarious discharges, especially nosebleed, and splitting headache. Congestion of ovaries; ovaries sensitive to touch. Whole abdomen painful at menstrual period. Threatened abortion from overexertion, overheating.

Painful inflammation of breasts, hardness at menstrual period. Rheumatic pain and swelling of the joints of the extremities. Joints are red, stiff.

Modalities: Worse: any motion, exertion, touch, warmth, warm food. Better: lying, especially on painful side; pressure; rest; cold; cold foods.

CALCAREA CARBONICA (*Calcarea ostrearum*, Calcium carbonate, Oystershell)
(kăl-kā're-a kär-bŏn'ĭ-ka)

Identification: *Calcarea carbonica* is an impure calcium carbonate that was first prepared by Hahnemann from oyster shells. The pure white portion of the shell between the interior and exterior surfaces is washed, dried, and reduced to fine powder. The lower potencies must be prepared by trituration.

Drug Action and History: Calcium is the fifth most abundant element in the human body, having a major function in the body structure and in maintaining the structural integrity of cells in multicellular membranes. Pathological conditions arising from abnormalities of calcium metabolism indicate that it plays a role in regulating the permeability of cell membranes to sodium and potassium. Abnormal blood calcium levels are associated with changes in the threshold of excitability of nervous and muscle tissue; decreased calcium levels, for example, are associated with decreased threshold to seizure activity. Hahnemann introduced *Calcarea* into homeopathic practice and described its symptom picture in *Chronic Diseases*. Nonhomeopaths have never considered calcium carbonate of much therapeutic value; at present calcium carbonate is a common allopathic antacid, but it has the drawback of producing acid rebound in the stomach.

Symptoms and Uses: *Calcarea* is a great constitutional remedy, one of the deepest-acting antipsorics. Its symptoms reflect impaired nutrition in the vegetative sphere. The *Calcarea* patient is usually pale, plump, flabby. *Calcarea* is a great children's remedy; children who grow fat, with large belly, large head, pale, or red-faced. Patients who are unable to assimilate calcium from their food become fat and flabby, with deficient bones; a high potency of *Calcarea* can reportedly restore the ability to assimilate lime. There is a lack of endurance, inability to rebound in both the physical and the mental spheres. *Calcarea* is full of congestive complaints, with blood rushing to the head, cold feet, congested chest. Congested parts become cold. Tissues are relaxed; muscles, veins, walls of blood vessels. Glandular swelling, hardness, soreness. Indurated ulcers. Abscesses in deep muscles; *Calcarea* will make the abscesses resorb without breaking. Exostoses from irregular distribution of lime. Softening and defective formation of bone. Children who are late to walk because of defective bones. *Calcarea* is an important remedy in rheumatic conditions of the joints. The *Calcarea* patient is chilly, sensitive to cold, change of weather. Increased sweat, in spots and generally.

Like the oyster from which it is derived, *Calcarea* reflects a soft, vulnerable inner organism that is walled off by a hard outer shell. The mental symptoms are marked by passivity, immobility, standstill, an ingoing state. The *Calcarea* patient shows a childlike vulnerability. Inability to sustain mental effort. He feels his weakness of mind and fears others are able to observe it. Broods over little things, little ideas, engages in petty activities. The *Calcarea* patient when healthy is a slow, conscientious worker; works well on his own, does not like to be given directions by others. When under stress from overwork in his business, he may give it up and sit at home. Indolence. The withdrawn mental state may lead to stubbornness, obstinacy.

Head sweats on slightest exertion; wets the pillow at night. Congestive headaches with cold head, better from hot applications. Recurrent constitutional headaches, occurring every seven or fourteen days, often brought on from exposure to cold. Slow formation of bones of skull; fontanels stay open a long time. Vertigo with cold head. The face is pale, covered with sweat. Painful swelling of glands of neck. Eye problems, with photophobia, worse from exertion, reading, writing. Dim vision; cataract, eyestrain. Weakness of eye muscles. Continually taking cold; chronic sore throat. Delayed dentition. Polyps of nose. Slow action of stomach; food doesn't digest, turns sour; sour eructations, vomit. Craving for eggs. Eats indigestible things—chalk, coal, wood. Swollen, hard, painful lymphatic glands in the abdomen. Sour, whitish stools. Sexual weakness; lassitude, sweating, weakness after intercourse. In the female, relaxation of the sexual organs. Warts and polypoid growths. Menses too early, last too long, profuse. Colds settle in chest. Painless hoarseness; weakness of vocal cords. Shortness of breath from slightest exertion. *Calcarea* encysts tubercular deposits; incipient phthisis. Weakness of the circulation. Palpitations. Vertigo from poor circulation. Rheumatic conditions of the joints, brought on by exposure to cold and damp. Feet cold and sweaty. Clumsiness, awkwardness, stiffness, weakness of the extremities. Weak spine; cannot sit upright, slides back in chair. Curvature of the spine. Sour odor of whole body. Profuse perspiration upper part of body.

Modalities: Worse: exertion, mental or physical, cold in every form, washing, moist air, wet weather, during full moon. Better: dry climate and weather, lying on painful side.

Relationships: Complementary: *Belladonna, Rhus tox., Lycopodium*, Silicea. Sulfur should not be given after *Calcarea*; *Calcarea* may follow sulfur.

CANTHARIS (Spanish Fly, Oil Beetle, Blister Beetle) (kăn'tha-rĭs)

Identification: *Cantharis* is derived from the bronze-green beetle *Cantharis vesicatoria*, commonly known as Spanish fly. The insect has a strong, disagreeable odor. The medicine is usually extracted with ether, using the whole insect; reportedly it takes nearly 13,000 dried insects to weigh one kilogram.

Drug Action: The blistering action of *Cantharis* is due to cantharidin, which acts on the skin and mucous membranes. The irritant action causes the capillaries to dilate and become more permeable; plasma escapes into the extracellular spaces, and as fluid collects under the epidermis, blisters form.

History: For centuries, Spanish fly has been popularly known as an aphrodisiac, deriving its reputation from its ability to irritate the mucous membranes, particularly of the urinary tract and sex organs. Its dangers are equally well known, and many deaths from Spanish fly have been reported. During the era of "heroic medicine," the substance was used as an external application to produce blistering. From the early eighteenth century on, it was used as a diuretic and as a remedy for blockage or retention of urine. Homeopaths extended this use of *Cantharis* to include kidney diseases as well. Contemporary allopathic preparations containing cantharidin are used topically for warts.

Symptoms and Uses: Characteristic of *Cantharis* is its ability to produce inflammation that leads rapidly to gangrene. The remedy has a particular affinity for the urinary and genital systems. All its symptoms appear with great intensity and progress rapidly. Complaints are attended by a burning sensation.

The mental state is marked by frenzy, delirium, excitement, rage. Thoughts run to the inflamed parts, generally the bladder and genitals, and so there is marked sexual excitement, frenzy, and sexual content in the language, often of an unexpectedly coarse nature. Restlessness; the patient moves constantly. In profound states, there is stupor, confusion.

Sudden loss of consciousness, with red face. Pale, wretched, deathlike appearance of the face. Hot head. Violent, bursting, lancinating headaches; sensation of burning in the brain. Erysipelas of face with large blisters. Eyes burning, smarting. Yellow vision. Watery, bloody fluid from the eyes that excoriates the skin of the face. Burning in the mouth, pharynx, and throat. Great unquenchable thirst, with aversion to fluids. Difficulty in swallowing liquids. Inflammation of the entire gastrointestinal canal, with burning in the stomach, esophagus, and especially the lower bowel. Abdomen swollen and tympanitic. Cutting and stabbing pains in the abdomen. Aversion to everything—drink, food, tobacco. Worse from drinking coffee, which increases pain in the bladder and is vomited. Watery, bloody diarrhea, excoriating the skin. Intolerable, constant urge to urinate, whether bladder is full or empty; urination gives no relief. Urine burns like fire; patient moans and screams on passing a drop. Bloody urine. Stabbing pains in the bladder. Painful, violent erections; penis inflamed and sore. In the female, oversensitiveness of all sexual organs. Burning in vagina. Inflamed ovaries and uterus. Menses too early, profuse, black. Nymphomania. Inflammation of lungs, gangrenous. Burning sensation in lungs. Pleurisy with exudation. Pericarditis, with effusion. Pulse feeble and irregular; palpitations. Tearing feeling in limbs. Burning of soles of feet at night. Violent lancinating pains through the kidneys and back and loins. On the skin there is an erysipelatous rash that turns black; tendency to gangrene. Eruptions burn when touched. *Cantharis* is useful, both externally and internally, for scalds and burns, with rawness and smarting, that are relieved by cold applications and are followed by undue inflammation. Fever with cold hands and feet, cold sweat, burning soles of feet.

Modalities: Worse: touch, on urination, drinking cold water or coffee. Better: from rubbing.

CAUSTICUM (Tincture *acris sine kali*, Hahnemann's *Causticum*) (kaw'stĭ-kŭm)

Identification: *Causticum* is prepared according to Hahnemann's instructions. A piece of recently burned lime (calcium oxide) is immersed in distilled water, then allowed to dry; it becomes a powder. This is mixed with bisulfate of potash that has been exposed to a red heat, cooled and pulverized, then dissolved in boiling water. The mixture is heated in a retort and the liquid that distills over contains concentrated *causticum*, which has an astringent, burning taste on the back of the tongue and which promotes decomposition of animal substances on which it is placed. The composition and strength of *causticum* are uncertain; therefore, it must be made exactly according to Hahnemann's directions.

History: *Causticum* is peculiar to homeopathy; it was introduced into homeopathic practice by Hahnemann.

Symptoms and Uses: *Causticum* is a deep-acting remedy. It is suitable for complaints in old, broken-down constitutions suffering from chronic diseases; only occasionally is it used in acute diseases. For chronic rheumatic, arthritic, and paralytic problems; slow, progressive complaints with gradual decline of the economy, decreasing muscle power. Weakness leading to gradual paralysis of single parts, generally on the right side. Contractures of the muscles and tendons; tendons become shortened, limbs drawn up. Rheumatic muscles and joints with shriveling, tightness, deformity of joints. Tearing, paralytic, numbing pains and soreness that remain in one place for a long time. Pains are better with warmth, worse in dry weather. Rawness and soreness of the scalp, the mucous membranes of the respiratory tract, the lower digestive tract, and the urethra, vagina, and uterus. Thick gluey discharges from the mucous membranes. Convulsive symptoms, twitching, tremulousness.

Broken-down mental state; brain tired; confusion, weak memory. Hopelessness, anxiety, melancholy. Hysterical cramping. Nervous system extremely sensitive; starting, twitching, jerking. Fearful fancies; always anticipating some dreadful event. Thinking about complaints aggravates them. Intense sympathy for the suffering of others. Nervous and mental symptoms brought on from suppression of eruptions.

Scalp contracted, tight, like the contractures in other parts. Eruptions on the head and face which, when suppressed, bring on chorea, facial paralysis, headaches. Wry neck. Neuralgic pains of the face from exposure to cold, often accompanied by facial paralysis. Fissures about lips, wings of nose, corners of eyes. Paralysis of the muscles of the eye and of the optic nerve; drooping lids. Disturbances in vision. Colds settling in the ear, with copious earwax; noises and reverberations in the ear; deafness. Paralysis of the organs of speech. Tongue awkward at talking and chewing; bites tongue and cheeks when chewing. The thought, sight, and smell of food take away appetite. Thirsty; drink of cold water relieves many conditions. Sensation of lime slaking in stomach. Averse to sweets; desires beer, smoked meats, pungent foods. Paralytic weakness of the rectum, which fills up with hard feces that pass involuntarily and unnoticed. Fissures in anus. Paralytic conditions of the bladder, causing either retention or involuntary urination; unconscious of stream as it passes; urine escapes involuntarily on coughing, sneezing, in sleep.

Hoarseness; loss of voice from paralysis of vocal cords. Hard cough that racks the whole body. Chest full of mucus, with sensation of tightness, relieved if patient can only cough deep enough to get a little mucus up, but mucus tends to slip back. Drink of cold water relieves. Contracted tendons in the extremities; rheumatic, tearing pains in limbs, better with heat. Paralysis of single parts. Arthritic deformities of joints. Stiffness; rises from sitting or lying with difficulty. Children slow learning to walk. Pain and stiffness in the back. Skin tends to grow warts, develops fissures on slightest provocation.

Modalities: Worse: dry, cold winds; clear, fine weather; cold air. Better: damp, wet weather; warmth; heat of bed.

CHAMOMILLA (Chamomile, Ground Apple, Whit Plant, Feverfew) (kăm-o-mĭl'la)

Identification: *Matricaria chamomilla* is an annual herb of the family Compositae, common in waste and cultivated ground in temperate regions of the Old World. The stem is one to two feet high, and there are numerous branches. The ray flowers are white and the disc flowers yellow; the composite bloom is about half an inch wide. The tincture is prepared from the whole plant, when in flower.

History: Chamomile has been in extensive use as a domestic remedy for centuries. In herbal medicine, chamomile is used in small doses as a mild tonic; in large doses it is capable of acting as an emetic. A digestive aid. Flowers are applied externally in the form of a fomentation in cases of irritation or inflammation of the abdominal viscera and as a gentle incitant for ulcers. Hahnemann published the first homeopathic provings of *Chamomilla* in 1805.

Symptoms and Uses: *Chamomilla* is full of marked sensitiveness and irritability. The *Chamomilla* patient is extremely sensitive to pain; pains are better with heat, except for the teeth and jaws, which are better with cold. The pains and sufferings are better with passive motion, especially in children, who must be carried and petted constantly. Pain makes the patient angry, scolding. Most complaints are worse from

9:00 P.M. to midnight. Neuralgic pains with numbness. Can't keep still because of pain; tosses in bed. An especially useful remedy for teething in infants who are peevish, restless, colicky, and must be carried. *Chamomilla* is not a deep-acting remedy.

The mental symptoms are prominent, and whenever *Chamomilla* is the correct remedy, the characteristic irritability, peevishness, and restlessness will be present. This is a leading remedy for anger and for complaints brought on by fits of anger from being contradicted. The *Chamomilla* child is crying, moaning piteously; he wants something new every minute, then refuses everything he has asked for. *Chamomilla* is not the correct remedy if a child is good-natured. Convulsions in children, often brought on by anger. When not in pain, the patient is melancholy, introspective.

Headaches in sensitive people, worse when thinking about their sufferings, better when occupied with other things. Face red and hot on one side, pale and cold on the other side. Toothache, better with cold, worse with heat. Very sensitive hearing; noises in ear. Severe earache, better with heat. Ears sensitive to wind. Great thirst for cold drinks, averse to warm drinks; averse to coffee, which makes the patient nauseous. Antidotes the effects of overuse of coffee. Colic in infants, with pain in stomach and abdomen; wind colic. Stools hot, green, slimy; diarrhea, with colic and with teething. Stools have smell of rotten eggs. In the female, profuse, clotted dark menses with laborlike pains. Menstrual cramps from anger, any excitement that irritates. Irregular contractions in labor, with irritability, scolding. Hard, dry, hacking cough; child coughs in his sleep. Coughing spells brought on by anger. Cough, chest complaints, laryngeal complaints generally worse at night. Pains in the extremities, followed by a feeling of numbness. Rheumatic pains that drive the patient out of bed at night; must walk about. Convulsions of the extremities. Burning of soles of feet at night; patient puts feet out of bed. Sleepless and restless during the first part of the night. Frightening dreams.

Modalities: Worse: heat, anger, open air, wind, night. Better: from being carried; warm, wet weather.

HEPAR SULPHURIS CALCAREUM (Impure Calcium Sulphide; Hepar Sulfur)
(hē'pär sŭl'fŭ-rĭs kăl-kā're-ŭm)

Identification: *Hepar sulphuris calcareum* (*Hepar sulph.*) is an impure calcium sulphide that was prepared originally by Hahnemann. It is still made according to his instructions, which involve heating finely powdered oystershell (impure calcium carbonate) and flowers of sulfur (sublimed sulfur) in a hermetically closed crucible. *Hepar sulph.* may take either of two forms: white porous friable masses, or a white amorphous powder. It is insoluble in water and alcohol and soluble in hot hydrochloric acid. The lower potencies are prepared by trituration.

Symptoms and Uses: The patient who needs *Hepar sulph.* is very chilly; all complaints are worse from cold. Complaints are aggravated by putting the hand or foot out from under the covers. Wears overcoat in warm weather. The *Hepar* patient is oversensitive and irritable, both mentally and physically, to surroundings, impressions, pain. Faints with the slightest pain. The pains of *Hepar sulph.* have a characteristic sharp, jagging quality, a sticking sensation like a splinter in the affected part. Another prominent feature of *Hepar sulph.* is that it promotes suppuration (the formation and discharge of pus); there may first be the characteristic sticking sensation, followed by a discharge of pus from the affected part. Tends to have skin eruptions and glandular swellings; lymphatic glands hard, enlarged. Offensive discharges, with a characteristic smell of old cheese; sour discharges; sour-smelling babies. Catarrhal state of mucous membranes, especially in the nose, ears, throat, larynx, chest. Sweats easily.

The mental symptoms are marked by *Hepar's* irritability; every little thing disturbs, makes the patient angry, abusive. Sudden impulses to do violence and to destroy. Quarrelsome; nothing pleases. Desires constant change, then is displeased by each new thing.

The *Hepar* patient is subject to coryza, with colds settling in the nose. Discharge is at first watery, then becomes thick, yellow, and offensive. Sneezing and running nose on going into a cold wind. Catarrhal affections of the ears, with sticking, tearing pains. Abscess in the ear; discharge with smell of old cheese. In the eyes, offensive, thick purulent discharges; inflammation of the eyes with small ulcers. Sore throat, sensitive to touch, with sensation of a fish bone or stick in the throat; sensation of a splinter on swallowing. Craving for sour and strong-tasting foods—acids, wine, spicy food. Stitching pain in the region of the liver on coughing, walking, breathing, touching. Catarrh of the bladder with purulent urine and mucopurulent deposits. Ulcers of bladder. Urine passes in a slow stream or in drops, with no force; in the male the urine drops perpendicularly. Sensation of a splinter in the urethra. Inflammatory strictures, with difficulty passing urine. In the male, suppuration of the inguinal glands. In the female, copious leukorrhea, with cheesy smell. *Hepar* has an affinity for the respiratory mucous membranes. Croupy, barking cough; cough brought on whenever any part of the body gets cold or uncovered. Larynx painful on talking, to touch. The patient becomes hoarse and loses voice with every exposure to cold, dry wind. At beginning of a cold, constriction in larynx that may extend up into the nose, down into the chest. The skin is very sensitive to touch. Ulcers, eruptions on the skin. Profuse sweat, sour, offensive. Abscesses; suppurating glands very sensitive. Every little injury suppurates. *Hepar* establishes suppuration around foreign bodies and so helps to dislodge splinters, projectiles, etc., that cannot be removed mechanically. Useful in felons when constitutional symptoms agree. In fever, sweating patient pulls covers around him.

Hepar is also used as an antidote to a state of mercurialization, with chilliness felt "in the bones"; sensitive to every change to cold weather, like a barometer. Useful in old cases of syphilis, especially when the symptoms have been suppressed by mercury. *Hepar* also has the fig warts of sycosis and chronic sycotic discharges with sensation of sticking in the ureter.

Because it promotes suppuration, *Hepar* must be used with great caution in cases where it would be dangerous for an old abscess to suppurate into a vital internal organ; high potencies must be avoided in old encysted tubercles in the lungs.

Modalities: Worse: dry, cold winds; cool air; slightest draft; touch; lying on painful side. Better: damp weather, wrapping head up, warmth, after eating.

Relationships: Follows mercury. The sequence of mercury-*Hepar*-Silicea is the proper order in which to administer these remedies; the cycle may then be repeated. Antidotes bad effects of mercury.

IGNATIA AMARA (Saint-Ignatius's-Bean)
(ĭg-nā'she-a a-mā'ra)

Identification: *Ignatia amara* is a shrub or tree of the family Loganiaceae. The tincture is prepared from the seed, or bean, of the pear-shaped fruit.

Drug Action: Saint Ignatius's bean contains strychnine, a virulent poison, in even greater quantity than *nux vomica,* but the provings develop important differences between the two remedies. (See *nux vomica* for a discussion of the drug action of strychnine.)

History: The Saint Ignatius's bean was named by the Jesuits, who in the seventeenth century introduced the seeds into Europe from the Philippines, where they were worn by the natives as amulets. Although *Ignatia* was in use in the seventeenth century, it was after Hahnemann published his provings of it in 1805 that use of the remedy was revived by homeopathy, largely for conditions similar to those indicating *nux vomica.*

Symptoms and Uses: *Ignatia* is particularly suited to sensitive, delicate constitutions; hysterical, overwrought women. The mental symptoms and central nervous symptoms predominate; hyperesthesia of all the senses; jerking, convulsive, twitching spasms. The remedy is full of erratic, contradictory, strange, rare, and peculiar symptoms. Although *Ignatia* and *Nux vomica* have many characteristics in common, *Ignatia* is reportedly more frequently called for in patients in the United States.

In the mental symptoms, the emotional element predominates. *Ignatia* is considered the principal remedy for grief. Hysteria. Effects of emotional shock. The patient is overwrought; from grief, from disappointment in love, from overapplication at school in science, music, or art. Misplaced affections. Hysterical debility and fainting fits; nervous, tremulous excitement, confusion. Changeable mood; introspective, silently brooding. Involuntary sighing. The *Ignatia* patient has strange antipathies; one cannot depend on her being reasonable.

In the head, pain like a nail sticking through the side of the head, better lying on painful side; congestive, pressing, tearing headache. All headaches better from heat. Headaches from abuse of coffee, tobacco, alcohol. Face distorted, convulsed, pale, sickly; pains in face. Face changes color at rest. Twitching of muscles of face and lips. Feeling of a lump in the throat that can't be swallowed. Sore throat, better from eating solids. Extreme aversion to tobacco smoke. Hysterical stomach; nausea, better from eating indigestible or acid things. Craves cold food; warm foods produce indigestion. With the characteristic mental state, a feeling of emptiness in the stomach and abdomen, with trembling. In the female, nervous troubles come on at the menstrual period. Much languor during menses. Dry, spasmodic cough; coughing increases the desire to cough rather than relieves. Jerking, quivering of the limbs. Inflamed joints, not painful to touch, sometimes better from pressure. In fevers, thirst during the chill, not during the fever. Chill not relieved by external heat. Itching during fever. Sleep very light; jerking of limbs on going to sleep. Insomnia from grief, anxieties.

Modalities: Worse: morning, open air, after meals, coffee, tobacco. Better: while eating, change of position.

Relationships: *Natrum muriaticum* is the chronic counterpart of *Ignatia* and often completes the case.

IPECACUANHA (Brown Ipecac Root, Brown Ipecac, Brazil Root)
(ĭp-e-kăk-yū-ăn′a)

Identification: *Ipecac* is derived from *Cephaelis ipecacuanha*, a shrubby perennial plant of the family Rubiaceae, native to Brazil and the upper part of South America, found in hot, moist forests, and cultivated in India and Malaysia. The plant has twisting, spreading roots, blackish green leaves, and very small white flowers. The tincture is prepared from the dried root.

History: The *Ipecac* root was long used by natives of Brazil as a treatment for diarrheas and was sold as a secret remedy to the French government in 1658. Its use in dysentery spread through Europe and India. The name in the vernacular means "vomit root," and was given to various roots; the botanical source was not identified until 1800. A nonhomeopath, Schoenheider, first mentioned the use of minute doses of *Ipecac* as an anti-emetic in 1791. In 1796, Hahnemann, applying the Law of Similars, reasoned that although *Ipecac* was generally known as an emetic, its use in minute quantities should cure nausea and vomiting. Hahnemann's provings were published in 1805. After *Ipecac* had been popularized as an anti-emetic by homeopathy, this use was taken up more generally in allopathy; at present, however, it is not employed for this purpose in orthodox medicine.

The active principles in *Ipecac* are emetine and cephaeline, both of which have amebecidal properties, with emetine the more active of the two. *Ipecac* has therefore been used in orthodox medicine to treat amebiasis. Although there are official preparations in the form of powder and syrup, *Ipecac* is rarely used today in orthodox medicine. It does have some limited use as an emetic and nauseant, and as a nauseant and expectorant in unproductive coughs. Syrup of *Ipecac* is given to produce vomiting in cases of oral ingestion of poisons.

Symptoms and Uses: *Ipecac* is used in acute illnesses where there is persistent nausea and vomiting, with nausea unrelieved by vomiting. It is associated with febrile conditions starting with pain in the back between the shoulders and extending down the back. The patient is usually thirstless.

Convulsions, spasmodic. Restlessness in spells. It is useful in patients with a hemorrhagic tendency; hemorrhages of bright red blood from the nose, uterus, kidneys, bowels, stomach, lungs. *Ipecac* symptoms come on rapidly, and it brings on the crisis quickly.

Pain in the back of the head and neck; congestive fullness in the head. Face flushed, bright red or bluish red, lips blue. Coryza in children or adults who catch cold in warm, moist weather, with stuffing up of the nose at night, sneezing, going on to hoarseness, rapidly spreading to the chest, the bronchial tubes. Nosebleeds with colds. Profuse saliva. All symptoms with nausea. Disordered stomach, sense of fullness, cutting pain spreading from left to right. Irritable stomach, gastritis. Constant nausea and vomiting. Vomiting of clots of blood. Epidemic and endemic dysentery; continuous urging with only a little slime or bright red stool; constant nausea. Dysenteric state in children with green slimy stool, vomiting of green curds. Pain in back in region of kidney. Urine contains blood and small clots. Uterine hemorrhages with profuse bright red blood, accompanied by nausea. Vomiting during pregnancy. Bronchitis in infants; they cough, gag, suffocate; coarse rattling in the chest; child looks pale, very sick, anxious. Old cases of asthma, with rattling, convulsive cough, gagging. Bleeding from lungs, with nausea. Effects of suppressed skin eruptions: acute stomach and bowel symptoms, colds settling in the chest. Symptoms from suppressed rash of measles, with nausea and vomiting.

Modalities: Worse: moist, warm wind; winter and dry weather; slightest motion.

LACHESIS (Venom of Surucucu or Bushmaster)
(lăk′e-sĭs)

Identification: This fascinating remedy is derived from the venom of a South American serpent, supposed to be the *Trigonocephalus lachesis,* commonly known as the bush master or surucucu. The exact species is in doubt. Potencies of the venom are prepared by trituration or dilution.

Drug Action: Serpent poisons kill by their effect on the nervous mechanisms of the heart. If death is delayed or if the dose is small, there are other effects, including local action on the blood, decreasing its coagulability and destroying the red corpuscles with extravasation under the skin. Lachesis has both these effects to a marked degree.

History: Constantine Hering was the first and principal prover of *Lachesis*, collecting it from the living snake during his stay in Dutch Guiana. He stunned the snake with a blow and expressed the poison onto sugar. In the process he absorbed some of the venom and experienced an accidental proving; when he recovered, his wife related all the symptoms he had exhibited.

The snake is a familiar•symbol that runs through the world's mythology, generally representing the primordial life energy, a hunger for life and knowledge, libido—the instinctual urges that are suppressed with the development of ego and the demands of civilization.

Symptoms and Uses: The symbolic significance of the snake interestingly finds expression in the symptoms from the provings. Complaints are predominantly left-sided, or begin on the left and spread to the right; compare this with the association of the left side of the body with the unconscious, with feeling and emotion. Similarly, the *Lachesis* patient sleeps into an aggravation; symptoms begin on entering sleep and increase as sleep progresses, so that on awaking the symptoms are most marked. Again, this corresponds with the taking over of unconscious impulses that are suppressed during waking hours but can invade the patient during sleep. Complaints are generally relieved by the appearance of discharges. There are constrictive sensations, corresponding to the blockage of vital energy and body fluids. The *Lachesis* patient cannot bear anything tight, particularly about the neck and waist. *Lachesis* is especially suited to patients of middle age and above, and it is useful in many complaints arising with the crisis of menopause. Reflecting its action on the blood, *Lachesis* is a hemorrhagic remedy; parts bleed easily, and there is bluish discoloration of parts. The blood when dried looks like charred straw or becomes black. *Lachesis* is a long-acting remedy; overdosing may poison the patient for a lifetime.

The mental symptoms reflect the symbolic interpretation of the snake. There is a dualistic sort of awareness and an intense awareness of the libidinous impulses that the patient has repressed; knowledge untasted, the penalty of a life unlived. Self-consciousness, conceit, envy, hatred, revenge, cruelty. Jealousy without reason, suspicion. The *Lachesis* patient is loquacious; impelled to talk continuously, jumping from one subject to another; can be witty and trenchant. There may be a paresis of the tongue, with thick speech, stumbling, as if intoxicated.

Head hot. Headache on waking. Surging headache in waves. Migraine. Vertigo. Head symptoms relieved by onset of discharge. The face reflects anxiety, distress. The skin of the face is mottled, purplish, puffed, or pale. Choking sensation; cannot bear a collar around the neck. Tongue swollen, trembling. Nasal catarrh, which sometimes relieves the headache. Gums swollen and spongy, bleed easily. Stringy saliva. Throat is dry, worse on left side or spreading from left to right; worse from swallowing liquids or empty swallowing; swallowing solids relieves. Abdomen distended, tympanitic. Liver region sensitive; jaundice. Cannot tolerate clothing about the waist. In the female, *Lachesis* has an affinity for the ovaries, particularly the left, or spreading from left to right. Menopausal symptoms; flushes of heat, rush of blood to head, disturbances of circulation, palpitations. Posthysterectomy symptoms. Menstrual difficulties, better during menstrual flow, worse before and after menses. Black menstrual discharge. Pain in the heart; signs of weakness of the heart, feeble pulse, difficult breathing. Enlargement of veins; sluggish circulation. Cold hands and feet from slightest exertion or emotion. Skin mottled, purplish, bluish; tendency to ulceration, bleeding black blood. Small wounds bleed much. Eruptions bleed easily.

Modalities: Worse: after sleep—sleeps into aggravation, left side, spring, pressure or constriction. Better: appearance of discharges.

LYCOPODIUM CLAVATUM (Club Moss, Wolf's Foot, Staghorn, Vegetable Sulphur)
(lī-ko-pō'dĭ-um kla-vā'tŭm)

Identification: *Lycopodium clavatum* is an evergreen trailing plant of the family Lycopodiaceae. The roots consist of strong fibers resembling a wolf's foot; hence the Latin name. The plant is very slow growing and matures slowly. The bloom is brown, in erect spikes, composed of an axis and many closely packed scales. On the scales are one-celled spores that look like a pale yellow powder. The spores float on water and are not wet by it. The remedy is prepared from the spores, preferably by long, laborious trituration; the spores must be thoroughly crushed to obtain the oil they contain.

History: Ancient physicians used the whole *Lycopodium* plant as a stomachic and diuretic, and the spores have been used internally for a variety of conditions. Externally, the spores were used as dusting powder in skin diseases and for chafing in infants. In the pharmacy, it is the best powder for keeping pills from sticking together. *Lycopodium* spores are highly flammable and are used in pyrotechnics. Although Hahnemann found *Lycopodium* already in use, particularly as a drying agent for pills, when he published his proving in 1828, it was generally believed that *Lycopodium* was medicinally inert. Homeopaths believe that the medicinal virtues of the spores can only be released by crushing them and administering the remedy in potencies.

Symptoms and Uses: *Lycopodium* is a polychrest with antipsoric, antisyphilitic, and antisycotic properties. It is a broad- and deep-acting remedy, ultimately producing tissue changes in the soft tissues, blood vessels, bones, liver, heart, and joints. It is particularly suited to individuals of keen intellect and weak muscular power, with dark complexions and dryness of the skin and mucous membranes. The symptoms are predominantly right-sided, or spreading from right to left, and from above downward. There is a characteristic pattern of emaciation from above downward, especially affecting the face, neck, and thorax, with the extremities well preserved. The patient is sensitive to cold, lacks vital heat. There is a characteristic aggravation of symptoms between 4:00 and 8:00 P.M. *Lycopodium* is an important remedy for gastrointestinal and liver disorders. The patient is full of gas. Premature aging.

The mental symptoms of *Lycopodium* come on gradually. The *Lycopodium* patient may appear extroverted, capable, but with a peculiar detachment, a sense of his own superiority. He may be a professional person whose work is largely intellectual. With the slightest suggestion of illness, he becomes hypochondriacal, headstrong, and haughty. As he enters middle age, or as he becomes ill, he develops a loss of self-confidence; dread of speaking in public when confronted with his audience. Failing brain power, indecision. Averse to company, yet dreads solitude; wants someone in the adjacent room. Sadness and gloom, better moving about a while. Psychosomatic ailments, particularly gastrointestinal.

Periodical headaches; headaches connected with gastric troubles. Headache from missing a meal. Premature baldness and graying of hair. Withered appearance of face, furrowing of brow, eyebrows drawn together, reflecting anxiety. Sensitive to impressions; twitching about the face when disturbed. Glandular swellings, suppuration, especially glands under the jaw. Chronic stuffiness of nose, with thick catarrhal discharge; head symptoms are better with discharge. Sore throat, tonsillitis, worse on right, or moving from right to left. Weakness of digestion. Gassy from least amount of food. Early satiety; the first mouthful fills him up. Bloated feeling. Rumbling of flatus, as if fermentation going on in the stomach; everything eaten turns to wind. Momentary relief with belching, but abdomen remains distended. Stomach better with warm drinks. Pain in liver; hepatitis. Inactivity of intestinal canal. Inactivity of bladder; must wait a long time for urine to pass, then it passes in a slow stream. Red sand in urine; when red sand present, head symptoms and chronic complaints are better. Frequency of urination at night, normal in daytime. In the male, impotence with a psychological overlay, lack of confidence; impotence from sexual excess. Right-sided hernia. In the female, inflammation, neuralgic pain in the ovaries, especially the right. Dryness of the vagina; pain on intercourse. Colds settle in the nose but generally move down into the chest; right lung affected more than left. Catarrh of chest with rattling, especially in infants. Shortness of breath, asthmatic breathing with chest catarrh. In grave respiratory illnesses, flapping of the wings of the nostrils. Gouty state of the extremities, better when red sand present in urine. Drawing and tearing pains in limbs, especially at night or at rest. Restlessness of the lower limbs, preventing sleep until midnight. Numbness of limbs. One foot hot, the other cold. Skin eruptions, ulcerations, hives with violent itching. Eczema in infants. Brown spots. Skin dry and shrunken.

Modalities: Worse: right side, above downward, 4:00 to 8:00 P.M., external heat. Better: motion, after midnight, warm food and drink, external cold.

Relationships: Follows sulphur and *Calcarea*.

MERCURIUS (Mercury, Quicksilver)
(mer-kū′rĭ-ŭs)

Identification: Two forms of mercury are used in homeopathy: *Mercurius vivus*, or elemental mercury, a silver liquid metal that is found in nature; and *Mercurius solubilis*, a powdered impure oxide of mercury prepared according to Hahnemann's formula from his prehomeopathic days. The symptoms for the two forms are virtually identical. Mercury is prepared by trituration in the lower potencies.

Drug Action: Although mercury, in its elemental form, passes through the digestive tract without being absorbed and therefore produces only temporary symptoms of distress, in various compounds, it is extremely toxic. It forms covalent bonds with sulfur, inactivating sulfhydryl enzymes and thereby interfering with cellular metabolism and function.

History: Mercury has a long history in medicine, owing to the ability of mercury compounds to promote secretions, including salivation and perspiration—two elements of "heroic medicine." Mercury was long used as a specific in the treatment of syphilis. In Hahnemann's time, the effects of poisoning from overdosing with mercury were well known. Complex organic mercury compounds have been used more recently in orthodox medicine as diuretics, and certain compounds of mercury are currently used in antiseptics, as parasiticides and fungicides for external application. Because mercury is an ingredient of commercial herbicides, fungicides, and water-base paints, accidental poisoning remains a problem today.

Symptoms and Uses: Hahnemann considered mercury the principal remedy for chronic syphilis, and many of mercury's symptoms resemble the symptoms of the secondary stage of syphilis, as well as the symptoms of overdosing with mercury that were common in his day. It produces catarrhal inflammations of the mucous membranes, with fetid, offensive, excoriating discharges. The mercury patient is sensitive to both heat and cold, remindful of the use of mercury to measure temperature. In general, the mercury patient exhibits weak reactive power in the face of stress. Rheumatic conditions of the joints. Bone pains. Inflamed, swollen glands. Tendency to ulceration and the foration of pus. Profuse sweating, which aggravates symptoms. Weakness and trembling. Many symptoms are worse lying on the right side. Worse at night.

The mental symptoms include restlessness, anxiety, "softening of the brain," and sluggishness. Impulsive insanity, as in old syphilitics. Feeble will. Weak memory. Hurried, rapid speech. Volatile.

Chronic rheumatic headaches. Rheumatic pains and neuralgias of the scalp, affected by the weather. Periosteal pains, worse in cold, damp weather. Exostoses in old syphilitics. Whole exterior head painful to touch. Loss of hair. Breath fetid. Metallic taste in mouth. Tongue flabby, swollen, bearing the imprint of the teeth. Tongue clumsy, trembling. Eye complaints from cold settling in the eyes. All eye troubles with intense lacrimation; tears excoriate cheeks; worse after exposure to radiated heat of a fire. Photophobia. Stinking greenish discharge from ears. Thick greenish yellow acrid discharge from nose. Much sneezing. Pain and swelling, caries of nasal bones. Teeth black, decaying, loose; gums red and soft. Copious, fetid salivation. Sore throat; inflamed, dry, spongy mucous membranes; swallowing with pain and paralytic weakness; difficulty swallowing fluids. Intense thirst. Sour stomach. Liver troubles, worse lying on right side. Great variety of stools. Slimy, bloody stools, much straining; a feeling of "never-get-done." Urine burning, copious, smarting, bloody; frequent urging. Chancres on genitals. Burning, stinging in ovaries. Excoriating leukorrhea in women; parts raw, sore, inflamed, itching; worse at night. Morning sickness with profuse salivation. Colds travel downward in the respiratory tree, from nose to throat; rawness and scraping of larynx; raw, sore chest. Colds settle in the bronchial tubes. Dry, fatiguing cough; worse at night, worse lying on right side. Inflammatory, rheumatic problems in the joints. Trembling of extremities. Bone pain in the limbs; worse at night. Unhealthy, moist skin. Excessive perspiration, especially at night, with an offensive, penetrating odor; sweating gives no relief of symptoms. Moist, oozing eruptions. Violent itching of skin, worse from warmth of bed at night.

Modalities: Worse: night, sweating, damp weather, lying right side, warm room or bed.

NATRUM MURIATICUM (Sodium Chloride, Table Salt)
(nā′trŭm mū-rĭ-ăt′ĭ-kŭm)

Identification: Common salt, or *Natrum muriaticum* (*Natrum mur.*), is, next to water, the most widely distributed substance in nature. It is found in nature in the form of rock salt, and it is also extracted from seawater. Homeopathic potencies are prepared either as solutions in water or as triturations.

History: Although salt was used traditionally as a remedy in some diseases (e.g., malaria), it was generally considered medicinally inert until Hahnemann conducted his provings in the 1820s. Because of its great osmotic power, sodium chloride in solution is used in orthodox medicine to maintain replacements of deficits in extracellular body fluids. In alchemy, a salt is any solid substance that has freed itself from a solution or from union with soluble or combustible compounds;

symbolically, with its source in the sea, *Natrum. mur.* might be seen as the individual mind or ego emerging from the collective unconscious, or the source of all life, in the ocean.

Symptoms and Uses: *Natrum mur.* is a polychrest whose action is slow, deep, and long in duration. It is particularly suited to constitutional prescribing, although it also has its applications in acute complaints. *Natrum mur.*'s physical effects are found in problems of reduced assimilation: aversion to food; emaciation from above downward, most notable in the neck; intermittent fevers; weakness and exhaustion; blood disorders, including anemias and white cell disturbances; and disturbances in elimination, with retention of water and waste products. The *natrum mur.* patient is chilly and catches cold easily. There is a dryness of the mucous membranes, or there is a watery or egg-white catarrh.

In the mental symptoms we find a confirmation of the alchemical and archetypal imagery associated with salt. The *Natrum mur.* patient is introverted, solitary, as if going through a period of ego development that must be worked out in solitude. Gloominess, bleakness, hidden grief; unable to cry, or crying in secrecy. Broods over unpleasant things from the past; never forgets an injury. Emotional, disturbed by excitement, worse from noise, music. Self-righteous; argumentative. Hysterical weeping alternating with laughing; easy, explosive laughter that acts as a safety valve for his deeply introverted state of mind. Though he seems to long for companionship and sympathy, consolation aggravates his mental state, sometimes bringing on anger. Ill at ease and awkward in company. Unrequited affections bring on complaints; misplaced affections. Dreams of robbers.

Compressive headaches, as if head were in a vise; hammering, throbbing pains. Headaches with zigzag dazzling. Face looks sickly, greasy, sallow, with emaciation about the neck. Eczema around hairline. Fluent running nose, with thin watery discharge, like egg white, going on to stoppage of nose. Fever blisters about lips. *Natrum mur.* stops colds beginning with sneezing when other symptoms agree. Reduced powers of assimilation; slowed action of the bowels. Constipation.

Craves salt. Averse to breads, fats, slimy foods like oysters, rich foods. Patient feels better when fasting. Great thirst for cold water, which sometimes relieves complaints, but thirst is sometimes unquenchable. Slowed action of the bladder. Must wait a long time before urine will start; cannot pass urine in the presence of others. In the female, dryness of the vagina with pain during intercourse. Nervous trembling throughout the body, jerking of limbs. Aching along spine, better lying on something hard or pressing back against something hard. Disturbances of the activity of the skin; waxy, shiny, pale, greasy appearance. Skin dry, withered, shrunken. Intermittent fevers. Chill in the morning, between 9:00 and 11:00, not relieved by heat or piling on clothing, but better from cold drinks.

Modalities: Worse: noise, music, warm room, lying down, about 10:00 A.M., at seashore, mental exertion, consolation, heat, talking. Better: open air, cold bathing, going without regular meals, lying on right side.

Relationships: Complementary to *Apis, Sepia, Ignatia.*

NUX VOMICA (Poison Nut, Quaker Buttons)
(nŭx vŏm′ĭ-ka)

Identification: *Strychnos nux-vomica* is an evergreen tree, native to India and the East Indies, of the family Loganiaceae. The name poison nut, or *Nux Vomica*, refers to the seeds of the berry. Incidentally, the Latin *vomica* has nothing to do with "vomit"; it refers rather to a depression, or cavity, in the seed, attributed by legend to the digital imprint of the Creator. The tincture is prepared from the coarsely powdered seeds.

Drug Action: Active alkaloids in nux vomica include strychnine, a virulent poison (also found in *Ignatia*), and brucine, a closely related but less potent substance. The action of strychnine is well known; it excites all portions of the central nervous system through selective blockage of inhibition, resulting in exaggerated reflex effects. It is a powerful convulsant; in the later stages of strychnine poisoning, all voluntary muscles, including those of the face, are in full contraction. Respiration ceases owing to contraction of the diaphragm and thoracic and abdominal muscles, leading to death from medullary paralysis due to hypoxia. In the early stages of poisoning, the victim is conscious, with heightened perception of all stimuli. The Nux seed also contains copper, which, like strychnine, has convulsive properties.

History: Strychnine, derived from nux vomica, was first used in medicine by the Arabians, who described it about 1540. In sixteenth-century Germany it was used as a rat poison. To some extent it was used medicinally in Europe, as a tonic, for example, during the eighteenth century, but its use was extended considerably following the introduction of Nux through Hahnemann's provings published in 1805. Subsequently, allopathic physicians used strychnine for paralytic conditions. At present there are no recognized medicinal applications for strychnine in orthodox medicine.

Symptoms and Uses: Nux is one of the greatest of the polychrests, since its pathogenesis resembles so many conditions for which patients seek treatment. The nux patient is thin, spare, quick, nervous, irritable; given to mental work and attendant mental stress. Either out of licentiousness or simply in order to keep going, he turns to stimulants, late hours, debauchery. Nux antidotes the effects of overdrugging from allopathic medications, coffee, tea, and alcohol. It is often the first remedy for patients who have been dosed heavily with allopathic drugs, since no reliable symptoms can be obtained until these drug effects have been cleared up. Nux is a great gastrointestinal remedy and a hangover remedy. Nux is full of hysterical manifestations. Europeans often develop symptoms calling for nux in their hysterical complaints; and Americans more often need *Ignatia*. The nux patient is irritable, oversensitive to everything—odors, noise, light, the slightest draft—and full of paralytic conditions, spasmodic conditions, convulsions; the patient is conscious or semiconscious throughout the spasm, with heightened senses. Characteristic of nux are actions turned in the wrong direction, a sort of antiperistalsis.

Mentally, the Nux patient is irritable, oversensitive, touchy, never satisfied. Can't bear conversation; wishes to be alone. Quarrelsome, reproachful. Melancholy, with sudden destructive impulses; tears things up. Anxiety, despair, hypochondriasis; overreacts to every complaint.

Headache with vertigo. Neuralgic headaches. Headaches from sweating; in wine drinkers; from staying up at night; relieved by absolute quiet. Headache in sunshine. Most symptoms are better from heat, but head symptoms are worse from heat. Always taking cold; cold settles in nose, throat, chest, ears. Stuffy nose, especially at night, outdoors, or alternating nostrils. Sneezing caused by itching in nose. Photophobia, much worse in the morning. Hyperesthesia of the nerves of the ear; loud sounds are painful, angering the patient. Nausea from overeating. Many kinds of food disturb— worse from meat; craves stimulants, pungent, bitter, succulent things; loves fats, which he tolerates well. Disordered stomach. Nausea and vomiting with reversed action; must strain to vomit. Portal congestion. Hemorrhoids. Must strain to pass scanty stool; when he strains, there is a sense of forcing the stool back—"antiperistalsis." The more he strains, the harder it is to pass stool. Diarrhea alternating with constipation. Irritable bladder; spasmodic sphincter. Reversed action on urination; must strain to urinate. Renal colic. Results of sexual overindulgence in both sexes. The male breaks down, becomes impotent. In the female, menses too soon, too long, copious. Pains, cramps in uterus, better heat and pressure, worse draft or cold. Asthma; especially from every stomach disorder. Coryza every time the stomach is disordered. Convulsions of individual muscles or of the whole body. Cramps in calves and soles of feet. Muscular twitchings, spasms, weakness, trembling, paralysis. Drawing pains in extremities, sacrum, hips. Paralytic weakness; disordered activity of muscles and nerves. Backache, lumbar region. Must sit up to turn in bed. Skin extremely sensitive to touch and draft. Tendency to jaundice in all febrile states. Chills and fever. Must be covered up in hot, sweating stage of fever as well as in chilly stage. Sleeps by fits and starts; jerking of limbs on going to sleep and in sleep. Wakes at

3:00 A.M., cannot sleep until toward morning, then wakes wretched, tired; wants to sleep late in the morning.

Modalities: Worse: morning, mental exertion, after eating, touch, spices, stimulants, narcotics, dry weather, cold. Better: from nap if allowed to finish it; in evening; at rest; in damp, wet weather; with strong pressure.

Relationships: Nux is closely related to Sulphur, which often completes the case. Nux also antidotes the superficial effects of overaction of Sulphur.

PHOSPHORUS (White Phosphorus)
(fŏs'fo-rŭs)

Identification: There are two forms of phosphorus: a red granular, relatively nontoxic form, and a white or yellow waxy, highly poisonous form. It is the white phosphorus that is used in homeopathy. White phosphorus burns on contact with air and must be preserved under water. It is highly flammable and burns with a brilliant white flame. The tincture is prepared as a saturated solution in alcohol, with a concentration of about 1/667. White phosphorus is unique among the nonradioactive substances in that, in the slow process of oxidation, it spontaneously gives off light without heat.

Drug Action: Phosphorus is an essential element in the body structure, in bone and nerve tissue; it is connected with calcium metabolism, hence influences the formation of bones, the development of hyper- or hypothyroidism, and the utilization of vitamin D. In cases of accidental poisoning, phosphorus has a toxic action within the gastrointestinal tract, followed by injury to the liver, muscles, myocardium, kidney, and central nervous system. The vomitus after ingestion of phosphorus has a garlicky odor and is luminescent. With chronic poisoning there is necrosis of bone, cirrhosis, and kidney damage.

History: Phosphorus is an ancient remedy that fell out of use in the nineteenth century because of its highly poisonous qualities. Hahnemann proved *Phosphoric acid* in 1819 and reported on the symptoms produced by *Phosphorus* in *Chronic Diseases* (1828). In the late nineteenth century, allopaths were using phosphorus in ways first popularized by Hahnemann. Today the use of phosphorus in allopathic medicine is limited; sodium phosphate is used to diminish hypercalcemia. Phosphorus is also a component of commercial insecticides, rodent poisons, fireworks, and fertilizers.

Symptoms and Uses: Phosphorus is a polychrest particularly suited to tall, thin narrow-chested people, with fair, transparent skin and soft hair. Such people may have feeble constitutions; they have grown up slender and too rapidly. Phosphorus is associated with destructive metabolism, hemorrhagic constitutions, fatty degeneration of the liver, heart, and kidneys, and dropsical conditions. The muscles are flabby. Rheumatic stiffness of all the limbs, especially on beginning to move; drawing, tearing pains in affected parts. The *Phosphorus* patient is sensitive to cold, worse from cold and better from heat, except for the head and stomach, which are better from cold. Necrosis of the bones, especially the jaw. Glandular enlargement. Burning pains. Weakness going on to paralytic symptoms. Always tired. It is dangerous to give *Phosphorus* in very high potencies in certain incurable tubercular conditions; it is also dangerous to give it too low or too often, especially in tuberculosis.

The mental symptoms of *Phosphorus* are reminiscent of the self-luminous qualities of the metal. The *Phosphorus* patient is self-centered; wants to be the center of attention; extroverted. Aware of other people more through intuition than through perception. Quick perception. Fear of being alone; loves company; loquacious. Artistic, visionary. Lack of mental stamina; irritability of mind, prostration of mind after slight mental effort; changeable; easily enthused but unreliable. Sensitive to external impressions: light, odors, noise, touch. Apprehensive during thunderstorms; can sense when they are coming; makes many complaints worse. Easily vexed. Anxiety, fear something will happen; anxiety about health.

Congestive, throbbing headaches, better cold, worse heat. Exostoses of skull, with tearing pains. Vertigo, staggering as if intoxicated. Dandruff. Hair falls out in patches. The face is sickly, pale, sunken, haggard, anemic. Red spots on cheeks in hectic fever. Necrosis of lower jaw. Neuralgia of face involving the jaws, temples, teeth. Distortions in color vision. Paralytic conditions of the eyes. A peculiar type of deafness; unable to understand the human voice; difficult hearing as if the ears were covered. In the nose, catarrh; painful dryness; alternately running and stopped up. Lips, mouth, and throat dry. Sore mucous membranes. Great thirst for ice-cold drinks; water is vomited when it becomes warm in the stomach. Violent hunger; hungry soon after eating; desire for cold food. Many complaints better after eating. Nervous dyspepsia; gastritis, pain, nausea, vomiting, burning. Eructations of food. Stomach symptoms better from cold things, worse from warm things. Liver congestion, fullness, pain, hardness, with fatty degeneration. Jaundice. *Phosphorus* is a very useful liver remedy. Kidney diseases; fatty degeneration of the kidneys. In the male, violent sexual desire with frequent painful erections. Impotence after excessive excitement. Involuntary emissions. In the female, excessive sexual excitement, but lack of sensation in the vagina during intercourse, as if numb. Colds settle in the chest. Inflammation of the larynx with hoarseness; pain in larynx on talking. Constricted sensation in chest, feeling of heaviness. Chest complaints worse from cold air; cough on going from warm into cold air. Pneumonia, worse lying on left side. Threatened tuberculosis. Violent palpitations of the heart, with anxiety; worse with motion, worse lying on left side. Cardiac affections with thirst for very cold water. Weakness of the limbs after mental or physical exertion. Paralytic weakness, twitching, trembling. Cold hands and arms. Hands, arms, fingertips numb. Emaciation of extremities. Weakness of lower limbs; unsteady gait; restlessness of limbs. All symptoms in the extremities better from heat. Stiffness in the back, back of neck. Stiffness on rising. A broad remedy in diseases of the spine. Dry, scaly eruptions on the skin. Purple, yellow spots. Ulcers. Small wounds bleed much. Numbness, formication, itching of paralyzed parts. Restless sleep, starting in sleep. Sleeps on right side.

Modalities: Worse: physical or mental exertion, evening, warm food or drink, lying on left or painful side, during thunderstorm. Better: in dark, lying on right side, being rubbed or mesmerized, cold food and cold water, until it gets warm.

Relationships: Arsenic is complementary to *Phosphorus*.

PULSATILLA (Windflower, Pasqueflower, Meadow Anemone) (pŭl-sa-tĭl'la)

Identification: *Pulsatilla nigricans* is a perennial herb of the family Ranunculaceae. The plant stands three to five inches high and its pendulous bell-shaped flowers are dark violet to light blue. The plant is clothed with long, silky hairs. It grows in open fields and plains, in dry places. It is known as the windflower because its seeds are scattered by the wind, and as the pasqueflower because it blooms at Easter time. The tincture is prepared from the whole fresh plant, when in flower.

History: *Pulsatilla* was introduced into medicine in 1771 by Anton von Stoerck, who reported using it in eye diseases, paralysis, rheumatism, amenorrhea, melancholy, skin disorders, and other conditions. It fell into disuse until it was revived by Hahnemann, who published his provings in 1805. Homeopaths used the remedy in eye diseases, inflammations, uterine disorders, menstrual troubles, and gonorrhea, and by the end of the nineteenth century allopaths were using it for the same disorders, although they sometimes tried to avoid giving Hahnemann credit for the reintroduction of the medicine. It is virtually unknown to modern allopathic medicine.

Symptoms and Uses: *Pulsatilla* is one of the most frequently used polychrests in homeopathy. Homeopaths take great aesthetic delight in describing the constitutional type associated with this remedy. The *Pulsatilla* patient is mild, gentle, tearful, affectionate, yielding. The remedy is commonly associated with women, particularly blondes, and with plump, rosy children. Although it is often referred to as a "woman's remedy" because of its affinity for the female reproductive system, it is used equally for men who have the mild *Pulsatilla* disposition. *Pulsatilla* complaints are better in the open air, worse in a warm room, better from gentle motion, but worse if the patient exercises sufficiently to warm up. *Pulsatilla* produces a characteristic catarrh of the mucous membranes, with a thick, bland green yellow discharge; the only exception is the vaginal discharge, which excoriates. The *Pulsatilla* patient is warm and wears light clothing even in chilly weather. *Pulsatilla* has many complaints connected with weakness of the digestion and the stomach, and with menstrual disorders. The symptoms constantly change; pains shift from one location to another, but they change in location only, not in class of disease. Many symptoms are relieved by the onset of the menstrual flow. *Pulsatilla* has one-sided headaches, one-sided complaints in general.

The *Pulsatilla* patient is dependent, eager to please, highly emotional, sentimental. The mental symptoms are marked by mildness, tearfulness, sadness, religious melancholy. The patient likes sympathy and is sympathetic with others. Irritable; easily slighted, touchy. Changeable. Full of whims. Mental and nervous symptoms are worse after eating, worse in the evening.

Headache before or during menses, or associated with menstrual disorders. Perspiration on one side of head and face. Face red, as if in health; the *Pulsatilla* patient often seems to be overrating her symptoms because she appears healthy. Many eye symptoms; catarrhal affections of the eyes, with thick, bland yellow green discharge. Stys with thick discharge. *Pulsatilla* is an important remedy for advanced head colds that settle in the eyes and nose; loss of sense of smell in acute and chronic catarrhs. Nose stuffed up in the evening and in a warm room, copious flow in the morning and in the open air. Slow digestion; indigestion, with bloating and distention of the abdomen after eating, especially after fats and rich foods. Averse to warm food and drink, fatty foods. Mouth, throat, and stomach symptoms worse in the morning. Dry mouth, but seldom thirsty. Colic in infants from fatty foods; infants with gas, vomiting. Continually changing nature of stools; no two stools alike. Bowel symptoms are worse evening and night. In the male, swollen testicles with mumps. A very frequently indicated remedy in gonorrhea with thick yellow green discharge. Late menstrual periods; menses suppressed from getting the feet wet. Flow greater during the day. Menstrual colic. Useful in many symptoms during pregnancy and confinement; pains are feeble, irregular, changeable. Useful in hay fever; other symptoms relieved when hay fever is present. Catarrh of chest, respiratory organs, with bland, thick greenish expectoration; bronchitis, pneumonia. Dry cough in the evening, loose in the morning. Rheumatic pains in the extremities and spine, wandering from place to place; worse with rest, better during gentle motion. Late falling asleep, and sleeps soundly late into the morning. Sleeps on back with hands over head.

Modalities: Worse: heat; rich, fat food; toward evening; warm room; lying on left or painful side; allowing feet to hang down; wind. Better: open air; motion; cold applications; cold food and drinks, though not thirsty.

RHUS TOXICODENDRON (Poison Ivy)
rŭs tŏx-ĭ-ko-dĕn'drŏn)

Identification: *Rhus toxicodendron (Rhus tox.),* of the family Anacardiaceae, is the familiar poison ivy, a deciduous shrub. The whole plant has a resinous, milky, acrid juice which is extremely poisonous. The poison is more active during the night and in damp weather. The fresh leaves are used in preparing the tincture. In preparing the potencies, the bottles must be handled with great care, since the tincture poisons the skin.

History: *Rhus tox.* was first used as a medicine in 1798, when a French physician found a patient's herpetic eruption cured by accidental *Rhus* poisoning. He then used the plant to treat herpetic eruptions and palsy. Hahnemann published his provings of *Rhus tox.* in 1816; in a typhus epidemic in 1813 he had used mainly *Rhus tox.* and *Bryonia.* Allopathy gradually revived the use of *Rhus tox.* because of the homeopathic example, reporting good results in scarlet fever, rheumatism, skin diseases, paralysis, and other conditions. In contemporary allopathic medicine, use is limited to the employment of *Rhus tox.* antigen for desensitization shots in patients susceptible to poison ivy.

Symptoms and Uses: *Rhus tox.* affects the skin, mucous membranes, and fibrous tissue—joints, tendons, sheaths. Characteristic are rheumatic pains and stiffness. *Rhus tox.* is an important remedy for first aid to sprains and strains. Complaints come on in cold, damp weather or from the suppression of sweat by getting wet while perspiring. Symptoms are generally worse on beginning motion, better with continued motion and walking, with limbering up, but prolonged motion or exertion of any kind leads to exhaustion. Aching pains, bruised feeling over the body, restlessness. Numbness and paralytic weakness of limbs.

The mental symptoms resemble those of low typhoid types of fever: incoherent talking, anxiety, fear. Mental symptoms worse at night. Despondency. Inability to sustain mental effort. Thoughts of suicide, but does not have the courage to carry them through. Restlessness, cannot stay long in one position, especially at night.

The brain feels loose in the head, as if it struck against the skull on moving. Muscles of head sore. Periosteum of cranium sensitive to touch. Pressure sensation in skull bones as if screwed together. Rheumatic headaches brought on by exposure to cold, damp weather or suppression of head sweat. Erysipelatous rash of face, burning, with large blisters, becoming purple, pitting on pressure. Eczema of face. Rash begins on left side, extending to right. Stiffness of jaw, cracking on chewing. Inflammation of eyes from cold, damp weather or suppressed sweat. Eyes swollen shut. Pain in eyes, worse on moving eyeballs. Nose stopped up from every cold. Triangular red tip on tongue. Neck stiff; swelling of glands in neck. Dryness of mouth and throat with extreme, unquenchable thirst, but cold drinks produce chilliness, cough. Painful, difficult swallowing because of inflammation, constriction of throat. Dry, teasing cough. Craves oysters, cold milk, sweets;

averse to meat. Soreness of abdomen to touch; can't bear pressure, sensitive to clothing. Swelling and tenderness on pressure of liver, cannot lie on right lobe of liver. Inflammation, erysipelatous, of male genitals; eczema; edematous swelling. In the female, swelling of vulva, with intense itching; erysipelatous swelling of genitals, with some eruptions. Weakness of all pelvic muscles, prolapse of the uterus from straining or lifting. Period too soon, too profuse, too long. Acrid flow, excoriating parts. Overexertion produced menorrhagia. Suppression of menses from getting chilled, wet. General inflammation and abscesses of glands. With colds, the larynx is raw; hoarseness when first beginning to sing, better after a few notes or talking a while. Soreness in chest. Gets out of breath on exertion. Inflammation of lungs and pleura, with stitching pain and much fever, tending toward the typhoid state; aching in bones, restlessness, better with motion. Pneumonia of low typhoid type. Useful for influenza, beginning in the chest, spreading to the larynx with hoarseness, when other *Rhus tox.* symptoms are present. Heart weak, tremulous at rest, with palpitation. Hypertrophy of heart from overexertion. Numbness and lameness of left arm with heart disease. Rheumatic conditions of the extremities from suppression of sweat, from getting chilled. Stitching, pressing pains. Stiffness and lameness, worse on beginning to move, wears off after moving about. Better lying on something hard. Paralysis, with numbness of affected parts. Weakness in joints following sprains; follows *Arnica* well when there is weakness of tendons and muscular fibers. Inflammation of the skin, becoming erysipelatous, purple, pitting on pressure, with large blisters. Intolerable itching, tingling, burning eruptions. Hives resulting from getting wet, or during rheumatism or chills and fever; worse in cold air.

Modalities: Worse: cold, wet rainy weather; at night; during rest; lying on back or right side. Better: warmth; warm, dry weather; motion; change of position; moving affected parts.

SEPIA (Inky Juice of the Cuttlefish)
(Sē'pĭ-a)

Identification: Sepia is the dried brownish black ink of *Sepia officinalis*, a mollusk more commonly known as the cuttlefish. The liquid, which is excreted by the animal as a protective, camouflaging device, is contained in an oval pouch, about the size and shape of a grape. The cuttlefish ink is procured enclosed in this sac, in which it is dried. In dried form it is insoluble in water, but diffuses readily in it, precipitating slowly. The lower potencies of Sepia are prepared by long, laborious trituration; it is difficult to subdivide.

History: Sepia, introduced by Hahnemann, is unknown to medicine outside homeopathy, although it is said that some preparation of cuttlefish was used by ancient physicians. The Sepia pigment used by artists comes from the same source, but it is not fit for medicinal use. Sepia consists largely of melanin, an intermediary product of the adrenal glands; interestingly, the adrenals are associated with recessive sex characteristics—i.e., male characteristics in women, and vice versa—and the symptomatology of the remedy is full of reversals and distortions of the sex role.

Symptoms and Uses: Sepia is preeminently a female remedy, associated with tall, slim women with narrow pelvises; a build not well-suited for childbearing. The female reproductive system is one of the remedy's chief spheres of action. The Sepia patient is marked by weariness, muscular laxness and weakness, sallow complexion. The complaints are full of bearing-down sensations in the abdomen or pelvis. Symptoms are generally worse at the beginning of motion and better with more strenuous exercise, after "warming up." The Sepia patient is chilly, lacking in vital heat.

In the mental sphere, the Sepia patient seems to have lost her ability to feel natural love; no affection for family, no interest in occupation. In the Sepia patient there seems to be a smoldering discontent, a craving for independence from the responsibilities of home and family. Illness is accompanied by a dullness of intellect, indifference, which shows on the face. Hysterical condition, with weeping, sadness, gentleness; then becoming disagreeable, excitable, obstinate. Will not be opposed in her opinions. Undependable, makes errors;

says and does strange things. Weeps when telling symptoms. Must always be annoying others; relating grievances, sarcastic, insulting. Miserly. Worse in company but fears to be alone. Excitable condition of the nervous system; disturbed by noise, slam of door.

Headaches, better lying down, worse with ordinary motion, better with exercise. Hair is dull, falls out. Face is sallow or pale; yellowish saddle across nose and cheeks. Large yellowish blotchy freckles on face. The face looks smooth, rounded, flabby, without the sharp lines and angles of intellect. Prolonged catarrh of nose; thick green yellow crusts blown from nose or hawked through the mouth. Wining, nasal voice. Gnawing hunger, feeling of emptiness in stomach, sometimes not relieved by eating. Craves sour, spicy, bitter foods. Aversion to food; the smell of cooking makes her nauseous. Spoiled, sour stomach. Nausea, sinking feeling. Pain in stomach worse with vomiting. Feeling of relaxation and bearing down of the abdominal organs. Inflammation of liver, jaundice. Liver sore, painful, better lying on right side. Constipation or alternating diarrhea and constipation. Sense of fullness, like a lump, in the rectum after stools. Ineffectual urging at stool. Involuntary urination with coughing, sneezing, laughing, surprise, when mind diverted, during first sleep. Pain in kidneys and bladder with bearing-down sensation. In the male, aversion to the opposite sex; impotence. In the female, dragging down of the pelvic organs, relaxation, as if everything would fall out; must cross legs to prevent protrusion. Tendency to abort during first three months. Loss of sexual desire; averse to opposite sex. Menstrual irregularity. Menopausal symptoms in Sepia constitutions. Catarrhal conditions of the chest, with thick, tenacious yellow expectoration; violent cough, retching, gagging. Weakness in small of back; soreness of back, aching pains, better with hard pressure; sits in chair with a book behind small of back. The skin is sallow, waxy, anemic looking, mottled with yellow. Liver spots on face, chest, abdomen. Looks prematurely old. Eruptions, herpetic, vesicular, scaly, and indurated.

Modalities: Worse: gentle motion, before and during menses, during pregnancy, after eating, change of weather, afternoon and evening, dampness. Better: violent exercise, pressure, heat, drawing limbs up.

Relationships: Complementary to *Natrum muriaticum.*

SILICEA (Silicic Anhydride, Oxide of Silicon (SiO$_2$), Quartz, Rock Crystal, Pure Flint)
(sĭl-ĭsh'e-a)

Identification: This oxide of silicon is a white amorphous powder, odorless and tasteless, soluble in water and dilute acids except for hydrochloric acid. It is prepared in a number of ways; Hahnemann obtained it from mountain crystal that was exposed to red heat or from pure white sand that was washed with vinegar, mixed with sodium, melted, and cooled. A British method uses silica powder and sodium carbonate. The lower potencies are prepared as triturations.

History: Silicea is virtually unknown outside homeopathy, although both Paracelsus and Glauber reported using it, and it has had some use in the ancient Indian system of Ayurvedic medicine. Silicon is a widely distributed element and the chief constituent of the earth's crust. It is an essential element of the supporting structures of many plants, as in stalks of grain or grass. Normal body tissues contain only traces of the element, but it is a component of dental enamel, nails, hair, and connective tissues. Silicea was introduced into homeopathy by Hahnemann. It is generally considered medicinally inert outside homeopathic practice.

Symptoms and Uses: Silicea, or Silica, is largely prescribed as a constitutional remedy for chronic complaints that develop slowly, corresponding with Silica's slow action. The Silica patient is of a sluggish constitution, with complaints arising from imperfect assimilation, slow nutrition. He is very chilly and likes to be well wrapped up. Tired after any exertion, either mental or physical. Silica has the ability to produce inflammation about any fibrous deposit and suppurate it out, reabsorb it. Tendency to form hard, glossy scar tissue. Silica will ripen abscesses and boils, suppurate out old wens, indurations, fibroids; promotes expulsion of foreign bodies. Complaints arising from the suppression of discharges, suppressed sweat, especially of the feet. Periodic complaints.

Silica is the chronic counterpart of *Pulsatilla*, and in the mental characteristics we find the same mild, gentle, tearful disposition. The Silica patient is lacking in "grit," both mental and physical. Timid, shy. Lacks stamina. Dreads undertaking anything new; the inability is only imaginary, and once he has begun the unusual task he feared, he does it well. Precise, high-strung, overconscientious. Irritable when aroused; easily startled. Fear of pointed objects. Child is cross when spoken to.

Chronic headaches with nausea. Profuse cold, clammy head sweat. Vertigo with nausea. Spreading ulcers on scalp. Hardened, swollen glands, especially about neck, parotids. Face sweats on exertion; lower body remains virtually dry. Eye complaints with intense photophobia. Ulcers on cornea; abscesses, boils, stys; has cured cataract. Chronic thick, yellow offensive catarrh of ears. Abnormalities in hearing; roaring in ears; pistol-like report in ear as accumulated fluids escape, with return of hearing. Destruction of bones in ear, nasal bones. Perforated septum. Teeth break down, lose enamel surface. Inflammation and swelling of glands of neck. Silica breaks up tendency to recurring throat complaints, tonsillitis, inveterate sore throat. Stomach is weak; slow digestion. Colic, flatulence. Averse to warm food; wants cold food and drinks. Abdominal pain better from external heat. Constipation from inability of rectum to expel feces. Stool slips back. Fistula in anus. In the male, chronic painful inflammation and induration of testes. In the female, prostration of sexual functions. Hydrosalpinx and pyosalpinx. Cysts. Silica aborts threatened abscesses of breasts; or, if they form, opens them quickly. Chronic tendency of colds to settle in the chest, with asthmatic symptoms. Chest filled with mucus, rattling respirations. Threatened tuberculosis. Heals small abscesses in lung. Early stage phthisis. Later stages of pneumonia; slow recovery after pneumonia. Affections of cartilage; growths about joints, about fingers and toes. Bones in children become softer. Caries of shafts of long bones, heads of bones, cartilage. Rough, brittle, crippled nails; ingrown toenails. Icy cold feet with offensive sweat. Skin delicate, waxy, pale, anemic. Warty growth on skin, eruptions, abscesses. Every little injury suppurates. Heals old fistulous openings with indurated margins.

Modalities: Worse: new moon, from washing, during menses, uncovering, especially head, lying down, lying on left side, cold. Better: warmth, wrapping up head, summer, wet or humid weather.

Relationships: Chronic counterpart of *Pulsatilla*.

SULPHUR (Sulfur, Flowers of Sulfur, Sublimed Sulfur, Brimstone) (sŭl'fur)

Identification: The sulphur used in homeopathy is a fine yellow greenish gritty powder. Sulphur is widely distributed in nature, sparse in its elemental form and widely combined with other metals. It is an essential chemical constitutent of all living tissue maintaining cellular respiration. Sulfur is insoluble in water. It may be prepared for homeopathic use either by trituration or as a tincture, with a concentration of 1:5000, in strong alcohol.

History: Sulphur has a long history in medicine. In the *Odyssey*, Homer mentions burning sulfur to purify the air, and Hippocrates considered it an effective antidote against plague. It has had long use among the lay public as an intestinal antiseptic, as in the "spring cleansing" of the intestinal tract with sulfur and molasses, still prevalent in some places. Sulfur has had wide use in medicine in skin diseases, both internally and topically, and it was an important chemical constituent of sulfa drugs, among the first of the modern "wonder drugs." The popularity of sulfur springs, used in treating a wide variety of ailments, including skin diseases and rheumatic conditions, led Hahnemann to observe that many people were poisoned by overuse of sulfur.

Symptoms and Uses: Hahnemann considered Sulphur the great antipsoric remedy, associated not only with the skin complaints of psora, but also with the chronic conditions that arose from suppressed symptoms. Sulphur is a common remedy for patients who have few symptoms to prescribe on, for the latent condition of symptoms owing to underlying psora. In practice, homeopaths often find that Sulphur will stir the reactive force of the organism when well-indicated remedies fail to act in acute diseases; or it will complete the action of acute remedies when there are underlying chronic problems. Sulfur has a centrifugal action, bringing complaints to the surface. The Sulphur patient is generally lean, hungry, dyspeptic, with a red, dirty face; he walks stooped over. He has a marked unconcern for cleanliness and tidiness, and he may dress in old, ragged clothes, working day and night in the midst of disorder. Scholars; inventors. The Sulphur patient is nicknamed the "ragged philosopher." Children who have an astonishing tendency to get filthy. Odors of discharges are filthy: breath, stool, genitals, fetid discharges, and the patient is nauseated by his own odors. Discharges are excoriating. Great itching and burning with complaints. Many complaints are worse from becoming warm in bed. Craves the open air. Aggravations at night, noon, once a week. Worse from standing; must sit or keep moving. Worse from water; dreads a bath. Bad effects of vaccination. It is dangerous to give Sulphur when there are structural changes in vital organs, especially the lungs.

The mental symptoms are full of Sulphur's disorderly qualities: the patient may be an inventive genius, but he cannot carry ideas through to completion. Selfishness; materialistic; collects things and ideas, rattles off facts and statistics. Philosophical mania, monomania; preoccupied with strange, occult, abstract things. Reasons endlessly over unsolvable questions. Aversion to systematic work. Religion melancholy; preoccupied with thoughts about his own salvation. Delusions; thinks rags are beautiful. Children dread being washed.

Heat in the top of the head. Periodical headaches recurring every week or every two weeks, with red face. Itching of head. Venous stasis of the face; red lips and face; face dirty, sickly, flushes easily. Moist, scaly, itching eruptions, worse from warmth. Colds settle in the eyes; many eye symptoms worse from bathing eyes. Catarrhal state of the eyes and ears. Sounds in ears. Deafness. Catarrhal affections of the nose; smells his own catarrh, which has an offensive odor. Imagines foul smells. All catarrhal discharges are acrid and burning. The Sulphur patient is thirsty for much water. Hungry; has sinking, empty sensation in stomach one hour before usual mealtime; cannot go long without eating. Dyspeptic; can digest almost nothing and must live on the simplest sorts of food. Pain and fullness in stomach after eating. Flatulent; belching, distention, rumbling. Liver enlargement; jaundice. Gallstones. Diarrhea drives him out of bed early in morning. Offensive, sickening stool; stool burns while passing and chafes the parts it contacts. Also constipation; large, hard stools. Eruptions on the genitals, with itching. Genitals have an offensive odor. In the female, burning in the vagina, itching of vulva. Offensive, acrid leukorrhea, which causes itching and excoriation. Colds settle in the chest or nose. Catarrhal states that hang on a long time. Incompletely resolved chronic complaints from lung diseases. Shortness of breath on exertion. Burning sensation in chest. Rheumatic complaints of the extremities; stiff joints. Cold feet daytime; burning in the soles of the feet, must put them out of bed at night. Hot, sweaty hands. Pain in back on rising from sitting; must walk bent, can only straighten slowly after moving. Skin unhealthy, dry, rough, scaly. Boils. Skin looks dirty no matter how much he washes. Wounds heal slowly; slightest injury suppurates. Skin itches, burns after scratching, worse from water. All orifices of the body are very red.

Modalities: Worse: at rest, when standing, warmth of bed, washing, bathing, in morning, 11:00 A.M., night, alcohol, periodically. Better: warm, dry weather; lying on right side; drawing up affected limbs.

Relationships: Sulphur is often followed by *Calcarea*, then *Lycopodium*; the series may then be repeated. Sulfur follows most acute remedies well.

THUJA OCCIDENTALIS (Arborvitae, Tree of Life, White Cedar, False White Cedar)
(thū′ya ŏk-sĭ-dĕn-tā′lis)

Identification: *Thuja occidentalis*, or the arborvitae, is an evergreen tree, from twenty to fifty feet high, of the family Coniferae. It is found in swampy areas and on cool rocky banks. The wood is durable. The tincture is prepared from the fresh leaves and twigs.

History: *Thuja* was used by the Egyptians for embalming and employed in medicine for centuries in a variety of diseases, including intermittent fever, coughs, scurvy, rheumatism, gout, and dropsy. The leaves and twigs, boiled with lard, were made into a salve for muscular aches and pains. Hahnemann introduced the plant into homeopathy by his proving in 1819; *Thuja* was taken up to some extent in allopathy in the treatment of both venereal and nonvenereal warts.

Symptoms and Uses: *Thuja* was Hahnemann's great antisycotic remedy, used in the treatment of sycotic (chronic gonorrheal) cases and of complaints arising from the suppression of sycotic fig warts. The skin of the face of the *Thuja* patient has a characteristc waxy, shiny, greasy appearance, sickly looking, entering on cachexia, as in sycotic constitutions and cancerous cachexia. *Thuja* is particularly suited to various kinds of wartlike excrescences that are soft, pulpy, very sensitive, burning, itching, and bleeding easily; cauliflowerlike growths on the mucous membranes; spongy tumors. Such growths appear particularly on the skin and mucous membranes in the anogenital region. Growths resulting from chronic irritation by discharges. Secretions have peculiar odors—of fish brine, garlic, honey. *Thuja* is a useful remedy for the ill effects of vaccination; for patients who have never felt well since a vaccination, or those who have animal poisoning in history. Symptoms have a tendency to be left-sided. The patient is chilly and sweaty.

The patient shows mental irritability, jealousy, and quarrelsomeness, especially with members of family. Fixed ideas; fears the body will break because it is made of glass; thinks there is an animal in the abdomen. Confusion, rush of thoughts, especially at night. Often slow in speech. Errors in reading and writing.

Left-sided headache accompanied by mental symptoms. Characteristic greasy, waxy appearance of face. Loss of appetite. Inflammation of the bladder and urethra, nongonorrheal. Constant urging to urinate, frequent urination accompanies pain symptoms. Enuresis. Urethral diseases of sycotic character. There is a pungent odor from the genitals, particularly when fig warts are present. In the female, a stitching, tearing pain in the ovaries, especially the left, increasing as the menstrual flow continues. Warty excrescences of the vulva and perineum. Rheumatic complaints from suppressed gonorrhea. Unhealthy, waxy skin; pulpy, warty excrescences; polyps, warts. Excess hair. Copious sweat, with peculiar sweetish or garlicky odor; sweat profuse on first going to sleep.

Modalities: Worse: night; heat of bed; 3:00 A.M. and 3:00 P.M.; cold, damp air. Better: drawing up a limb.

7

CASE STUDIES

Case studies from the homeopathic literature illustrate the application of the homeopathic doctrine in practice and document some of the remarkable cures reported.

One of the problems with homeopathic case studies is that although cures may be copiously reported, failures are rarely documented. Isolated reports of cures do not in themselves prove that homeopathy works in all instances, any more than do such clinical reports by allopaths or other healers. Only carefully controlled studies can establish the scientific validity of cures that may be applicable to large populations. Remarkable individual cures are common throughout world medical literature, ranging from "miracles" effected by remote folk healers to the "cures" of highly technical medical practitioners. It is not the individual success stories that constitute medical breakthroughs; it is the effective elimination of disease and disorder among large populations using a designed medicine or method that we can safely term a cure.

The language of the homeopaths in some of the following case studies communicates the enthusiasm and dedication with which they apply Hahnemann's doctrine. Other cases are reported dryly in the language of conventional medical history. Sometimes laboratory findings are included, illustrating that homeopathic remedies are capable of influencing these objective diagnostic parameters. We have also included some comments on cases that are particularly illustrative of the homeopathic approach.

A CASE FROM HAHNEMANN

Samuel Hahnemann treated thousands of patients, but he published only two case histories in all his voluminous writings. The following is one of them, and it illustrates how Hahnemann matched the patient's symptoms to those of the proper remedy. There were no repertories in Hahnemann's time, and so he had to determine the *simillimum* on the basis of his own thorough familiarity with the actions of the remedies as demonstrated both in the provings and in his own practice.

In this case, apparently Hahnemann was still simply diluting the remedies in serial fashion, without succession, to avoid serious aggravations. He does not refer to the remedy as a potency, but rather as a "very minute dose."

W., a weakly pale man of 42, who was constantly kept by his business at his desk, had been ill five days. (December 27th, 1815.)

(a) The first evening he became, without manifest cause, sick and giddy with much eructation.

(b) 2 a.m. the following night, sour vomiting.

(c) Subsequent nights severe eructation.

(d) To-day also sick eructation of fetid and sour taste.

(e) Felt as if food lay crude and undigested in stomach.

(f) In head, vacant, hollow and confused, and as if sensitive therein.

(g) The least noise was painful to him.

(h) He is of a mild, soft, patient disposition.

Here I may observe:

To (a) That several medicines cause vertigo with nausea, as well as *Pulsatilla* (3),* which produces its vertigo in the evening also (7) a circumstance that has been observed from few others.

To (b) *Stramonium* and *Nux vomica* cause vomiting of sour and sour-smelling mucus, but, as far as is known, not at night. *Valerian* and *Cocculus* cause vomiting at night, but not of sour stuff. *Iron* alone causes vomiting at night (61,62), and can also cause sour vomiting, (66) but not the other symptoms observed.

Pulsatilla, however, causes not only sour vomiting in the evening (349,356) and a nocturnal vomiting in general, but also the other symptoms of this case not found among those of *Iron*.

* The figures refer to symptoms in Hahnemann's *Materia Medica Pura*.

To (c) Nocturnal eructation is peculiar to *Pulsatilla* (296, 297).

To (d) Fetid, putrid (259) and sour eructation (301, 302) are peculiar to *Pulsatilla*.

To (e) The sensation of indigestion of the food in the stomach is produced by few medicines, and by none in such perfect and striking manner as by *Pulsatilla* (321, 322, 327).

To (f) With the exception of *Ignatia* (2) which, however, cannot produce the other ailments, the same state is only produced by *Pulsatilla*. (39 compared with 40, 81.)

To (g) *Pulsatilla* produces the same state (995), and it also causes over-sensitiveness of other organs of the senses, for example of the sight (107). And although intolerance of noise is also met with in *Nux vomica*, *Ignatia* and *Aconite*, yet these medicines are not homoeopathic to the other symptoms and still less do they possess symptom (h), the mild character of the disposition, which, as stated in the preface to *Pulsatilla*, is particularly indicative of this plant.

The patient, therefore, could not be cured in a more easy, certain and permanent manner than by *Pulsatilla*, which was accordingly given to him immediately, but on account of his weakly and delicate state only in a very minute dose, i.e. half a drop of the quadrillionth of a strong drop of *Pulsatilla*. This was done in the evening.

The next day he was free of all ailments, his digestion was restored, and a week thereafter, as I was told by him, he remained free from complaint and quite well.

The investigation in such a slight case of disease, and the choice of the homoeopathic remedy for it, is *very speedily* effected by the practitioner who has had only a little experience in it, and who either has the symptoms of the medicine in his memory, or who knows where to find them readily; but to give in writing all the reasons *pro* and *con* (which would be perceived by the mind in a few seconds) gives rise, as we see, to tedious prolixity.

For the convenience of treatment, we require merely to indicate for each symptom all the medicines which can produce the same symptoms by a few letters (e.g. *Ferr.*, *Chin.*, *Puls.*) and also to bear in mind the circumstances under which they occur, that have a determining influence on our choice and in the same way with all the other symptoms, by what medicine each is excited, and from the list so prepared we shall be able to perceive which of the medicines homoeopathically covers the most of the symptoms present, especially the most peculiar and characteristic ones, and this is the remedy sought for.[1]

1. From Samuel Hahnemann, *Lesser Writings*, Quoted in *Homeotherapy* 4, no. 1 (February 1978): 6–7.

CASES FROM KENT

James Tyler Kent (1849–1916), considered one of the greatest homeopathic physicians, was the author of the monumental *Repertory of the Homoeopathic Materia Medica*—to this day the mainstay of homeopathic prescribers. In his teachings, Kent insisted on strict adherence to Hahnemann's principles; in his practice, he demonstrated the effectiveness of the very high potencies. Pure, classical homeopathy is frequently referred to as "Kentian" by modern homeopaths.

The first report below, a case of chronic arthritis, illustrates not only the selection of the remedy on the basis of the symptoms, but also the prescription of placebo, or *saccharum lactis* (*sac. lac.*), during periods when the remedy is continuing to work. The homeopathic aggravation is well documented in this case. In the course of treatment, Kent also prescribes an acute remedy, *Ignatia,* for aggravation of the chronic symptoms by grief. With changes of symptoms, Kent changes the prescription; the overall pattern is the sequence of *Sulfur-Calcarea-Lycopodium,* which is frequently observed in chronic cases. Since the remedies given are all covered in chapter 6, it is instructive to compare the indications in the case with the symptom pictures described in that chapter.

Mrs. N., age, about thirty-eight, has for about ten years been an invalid as a result of chronic arthritis of the left knee. When it was in the acute stage she was treated by Dr. Hammer, a well-known St. Louis surgeon. It was cupped and blistered but the disease progressed. She was treated by the best allopathic surgeons and still it progressed. The last to have control of it was our lamented Dr. Hodgen, who placed it in a splint, saying that if anchylosis could not be accomplished it must come off. "A stiff leg or no leg," was his language. Two months in a splint failed to accomplish anchylosis.

July 16, 1881, I was called to the case. The knee was painful and extremely sore to touch, enlarged to twice the size of the well one and very hard. The thigh was emaciated and the ankle and feet were oedematous. The limb was wrapped and she was in bed. She could sit up but the limb could not be moved much, it was so painful from motion. There was great burning in the soles and top of the head. Sulph. 55000 one dose dry. Sac. lac.

The husband came to me the next morning, saying that Mrs. N. was much worse. She had suffered greatly during the night and had pain all over the body. I visited her and urged her to bear her suffering, that it would pass off soon. She took Sac. Lac. till August 20th, and Sulph. 81m was given, one dose dry. Slight aggravation followed, but she said she could bear it, as the first medicine which aggravated had been followed by such relief. September 1st. The pain has all subsided and she is moving about the house on crutches. September 20th, she sent for me. I found crepe on the door and learned that her husband had been sick a week and had died under allopathic treatment; that she had been up night and day attending him and was very nervous and the limb was much more painful. She took Ignatia for some days until the sad occasion had passed over a little, when I again paid my attention to the knee. October 8th she took Sulph. 81m and she thought it gave her rest, but not much improvement in the knee. She continued Sac. Lac. to November 12th. The joint has grown smaller, the foot is not so oedematous, no burning in the soles or top of head. Her appetite is good and she is gaining strength. In a general way she is much improved. Not seeing how matters could be improved by medicine, without better indications, I concluded to continue Sac. Lac.

December 3d. She complained of cold feet and that every change in the weather from warm to cold gave her pain in the knee and she had a craving for eggs. She had difficulty in keeping warm. Calc. 85m and Sac. Lac. for a month.

January 7th, 1882—Feeling very comfortable; slept well most of her nights; feet warm, and there was not much pain in the knee; swelling in knee going down; she is about the house on crutches; the sensitiveness is gradually going out of the knee. Sac. Lac.

During all this time there has been limited motion in the limb, but the slightest motion has always caused pain, but she has been able to swing it off the bed, holding the foot up to prevent flexion and then with her crutches she has been going about the house with comparative comfort.

February 3d.—Calc. 85m. Improving slowly.

March 25th.—There is some motion in the knee without much pain; the joint is slowly growing smaller; no swelling of the foot; she now wears a shoe that mates the right, the first time for ten years or more. Sac. Lac.

April 4th.—No new symptoms; improvement has ceased. Calc-c. 85m and Sac. Lac.

May 3d.—No change from last date; no new symptoms; eating well, sleeping well; countenance looks well. What shall I do? Prescribe for the knee? No, I wait Sac. Lac.

June 3d.—Sour eructations that seem to burn the pharynx but do not come up into the mouth; knee more painful; nights restless; must move about, which seems to relieve; drawing pain in the knee; gnawing pain in the stomach. "A sour eructation, the taste of which does not remain in the mouth, but the acid gnaws in the stomach" Lyc. "Incomplete burning eructations which only rise into the pharynx, where they cause a burning for several hours" (Allen) Lyc.

Lycopodium having all the rest of the symptoms, it was given 71m, and Sac. Lac. The knee became very painful and she was compelled to keep her bed for several days. Each day I visited her and she took Sac. Lac.

July 2d.—She is walking with crutches and has very little pain in the knee; no pain in the stomach or eructation. Improving.

August 3d.—Improving. Sac. Lac.

September 2d.—Lycop. 71m and Sac. Lac.

September 6th.—Slight aggravation from the Lyc. Improving.

October 1st.—Improving. Sac. Lac.

November 8th.—Improving. Sac. Lac.

December 15th.—Lycopod. 71m and Sac. Lac.

January, 1883.—It is now eighteen months since taking this case. The patient is in good flesh, and the knee is the only thing that gives her trouble. There is still limited motion. The motion is not much painful except when forced flexion is attempted. She goes about the yard and out into the road. I furnished her a cane and advised laying aside one of the crutches. She has no fear of the knee being hit, which heretofore has been a great factor in the case.

May 1.—She walks with a crutch and cane. Limbs gaining motion continuously. No new symptoms, knee nearly natural. She can bear some weight on the left foot. Lyc. 71m dry and Sac. Lac.

July 8th.—Rheumatism pains in both knees and such restlessness that she moves all night. Stiffness in joints, which passes off by motion; while in motion she feels better, Rhus. tox. 1m in water every three hours.

July 10th.—Improved. Restlessness all gone. Stiffness some better. Sac. Lac.

August 5th.—Improving. Rhus. tox. 32m one dose, and Sac. Lac.

September 1st.—I found her walking with one cane. She moved over the house to show me how well she could walk.

October 1st.—Improving. Rhus. tox. 32m one dose, and Sac. Lac.

November 8th.—Rhus. tox. 32m one dose, and Sac. Lac.

December 5th.—She walked with the aid of her cane two blocks to a street car, and came to my office without the aid of the cane. January 7th., 1884.—Came to my office. She walks with a limp. Limited motion in the knee, but the soreness has gone. I asked her if she regretted going under constitutional treatment, to which she answered: "Ten thousand times, no."

I have referred to two distinguished allopathic attendants, simply to show that the best surgical skill had been applied, and that the value of the purely homoeopathic method may be better appreciated. Ten years she grew worse, and in two and one-half years she was cured. If it can be argued that she recovered without medicine, then the means that had been used were destroying her life.[2]

The next case is more acute in nature: a bubo, or enlarged and inflamed lymph node, with an associated chancre, a lesion occurring at the site of entry of infection. It is not clear whether the case is syphilitic in nature; no diagnostic name is ever applied. The remedy is one of the animal poisons, derived from the tarantula. The homeopathic aggravation brings out mental symptoms characteristic of the remedy, which was given in the 12x, or a dilution of 1/1,000,000,000,000—a relatively low potency!

Case I.—A young man came to me with a bubo in the left groin. He had been disappointed in that he had not obtained relief from the treatment used. His bones ached, his tongue was loaded, and his breath smelled badly. The tumifacation was hard and painful, *bluish and mottled, with great burning and sharp cutting pains*. It was discovered some distance around and the heat was intense. He took Tarantula cubensis 12x, and one powder dry on the tongue three mornings in succession. He returned on the third day after taking his last powder saying that he was poisoned. He complained of a wild feeling in his brain and a drawing sensation in the scalp and muscles of the face. He was in a great state of mental anxiety and said he felt as if he was going to lose his reason. Mental restlessness was marked in his countenance. He could not keep quiet even after I assured him that he was in no danger. His primary symptoms had nearly gone and the bubo had lost its bad color. The next day he was much improved in a general way and the bubo had nearly

2. J. T. Kent, A.M., M.D., *New Remedies, Clinical Cases, Lesser Writings, Aphorisms and Precepts* (New Delhi: B. Jain Publishers, 1976), pp. 535–38.

disappeared. I saw him again in three days and the improvement was going on rapidly. The chancre healed rapidly and in one month he told me he had never been so well.[3]

In the following case of mental illness, Kent illustrates the process of repertorization. Referring to the grades of the symptoms in his *Repertory*, a value of 3 is assigned to symptoms of the first grade (all capitals); 2 to the second grade (italics); and 1 to the third grade (lower case). Note that the violent mental symptoms are strongly related to the remedies containing the *belladonna* alkaloids—*Belladonna (Bell.), Hyoscyamus (Hyos.),* and stramonium *(stram.).* The symbols for the modalities ⟨for aggravation and⟩ for amelioration, are used in this report.

R.T., aged twenty-three years, had gonorrhoea which was treated allopathically for four months before it was controlled. Habits of secret vice. Was sent home from college for treatment.

Mental condition, diagnosed by a specialist "Dementia praecox"; Weeping; Forgets everything; Answers no questions, makes unintelligible, slight mumbling; Hears voices; Thinks he is a criminal; Thought he was Christ; Thought he was to be buried alive; Hears officers coming to arrest him; Mind appears to be gone; Hands and feet clammy. Violent—had to be tied and held in bed. Face red; continually flaming red. Head—pain in occiput ⟩ in middle of day. Ears—pressed-in sensation. Constipation. Wakens with a start. Noise ⟨ Light ⟩ L. pupil appears larger than right. Medor. 10. Given to test the case to determine if it were a case of suppressed sycosis. No response followed and the case was thus determined not due to suppression. Under observation day and night by day and night nurse.

Mar. 23. Hears voice from a distance: of father: of mother: of policeman. Voice called him a liar; voices said he was dead; told him to "run for it;" of mother, told him to say "Lord" very loud. Thinks he is damned; that people are laughing at him. Somewhat religious phases of delirium; commanded by one of the voices to say the Apostles' Creed. Breath fetid, ever since he came home, now better. Fecal evacuations were black when first returned home. Voices: Bell., cann.-ind., carb.-s., cinch., *cham.,* crot-c., *elaps.,* hyos., *kali-br.,* lach., lyc., med., phos., stram.; many more not related to him.

Religious affections: *Bell.,* carb.-s., *cham.,* HYOS., kali-br., LACH., *lyc., med., stram.*

3. Ibid., p. 522.

Weeps: *Bell.*, CARB-S., *cham.*, *hyos.*, KALI-BR., lach., LYC., *med.*, stram.
Mania: BELL., HYOS., KALI-BR., *lach.*, LYC., STRAM.
Insanity: BELL., HYOS., *kali-br.*, *lach.*, LUC., STRAM.
Answers incoherent: HYOS.
Irrelevant: *Hyos.*
Confused speech: Bell., *hyos.*, lach., med.
Incoherent speech: Bell., HYOS., kali-br., LACH., STRAM.
Confusion: BELL., *hyos.*, kali-br., *lach.*, med., stram.
Delirium: BELL., HYOS., kali-br., LACH., STRAM.
Delirium raving: BELL., HYOS., LYC., *stram.*
Chill: *Bell.*, *hyos.*, *lach.*, *stram.*
Summary: Bell. 24; Hyos. 27; Lach. 20; Stram. 21.
Hot head: Bell., hyos., lach., stram.
Cold feet: BELL., *hyos.*, LACH., STRAM.
Clothing ⟨*neck: Bell.*, LACH.
Occipital pain: BELL., *hyos.*, *lach.*, stram.
Starting on waking: BELL., HYOS., *stram.*
Light ⟨: *Bell.*, *hyos.*, *lach.*, *stram.*
Noise L⟩: BELL., hyos., *lach.*
Summary: Bell. 44; Hyos. 38; Stram. 34.

Though Bell. stands highest in the anamnesis, the bodily heat of the remedy is lacking and the case may later demand Hyos., as the mania is not active enough for Stram. Bell. 10m.

S.L. two hours in water.

Mar. 25. Struck his nose twice; Bell., hyos., stram. Thinks he is about to be arrested: Bell. Just ascertained that he has lost all shame. No other change. Hyos. 10m.

Mar. 26. Thinks his medicine is poison. Breath less offensive. Hears scarcely any noises. Sach. lact.

April 4. Voices say he is dead and he wants to know when they are going to have the funeral. Wants to dig his own grave. Wants to be buried. Thinks his coffin is in the house or cellar. Rubs his nose much, it itches. Thinks the medicine is poison. Collar fits too close. Lach. 10m.

April 9. Thought that he was dead only once; voices less. Feet and hands cold. Sach. lac.

April 12. Struck his attendant several times. Quarrelsome; wants to fight. Thinks he is a criminal. Appears worse on Lachesis. Hyos. 10m.

April 13. No more fighting since last remedy. More quiet; appearance improved; face less red; nose itches less; does not rub it constantly, as he did.

April 18. Laughs much. Hears voices of the family and of the nurse. Thinks he is a criminal. No initiative: waits for commands before action; when told to eat he eats; to go to bed, he goes to bed, stands until told to sit and sits until told to stand; when told to do anything he does it, almost mechanically. Irresolution. Does not talk; appears unable to answer. Sach. lac.

May 2. Heat in head marked;)by cold. Aversion to hot soup. Intense fear. Nervous. Voices. Delusions. Irresolution. Phos. 10m.

Remedies heretofore used removed the violence and the intensity of the mania, so that he could eat at the table with the family. He was constantly under the observation of a carefully observant nurse, who at this time noticed that he could not take hot soup. In connection with the other symptoms, it was evident that Phosphorus was closely related throughout the case. Hence the prescription.

May 28. Much improved; no delusions; seldom hears voices. Now very nervous. Aversion to being touched. Likes cold water. Phos. 10m.

This case was finished by a repetition of Phos. in 50m. potency, a month later. By the middle of June, the mental symptoms had disappeared and he had gained much flesh. Since that he has been normal and robust, traveling about the city as would any one else.[4]

The use of the nosode *tuberculinum* is illustrated in the following case. In the course of cure Kent observes that the symptoms move in the direction of Hering's law: as the glandular problem in the neck lessens, gouty problems appear in the extremities (from above downward; from more important to less important organs).

Dec. 30, 1907. Tubercular glands in left side of neck. These had been examined by allopaths and condemned to operative treatment. Very sensitive to warm room; must have fresh air at night. Feels well indoors or outside. Appetite good; bowels normal. Active, attends to her own housework. Feet cold; hands cold easily. Appearance of face, sickly; dull red color. Tuberc. 10m.

Jan. 27, 1908. Had a cold she called Grippe, two weeks ago, cured with Ars. 10m. Tuberc. 10m. Repeated also Feb. 24.

Apr. 6. Gland in left side neck began to be sore about three days ago. Remedy acted over forty days. Tuberc. 50m.

Apr. 21. Swelling of lump continued a week, with some suppuration; two days ago began to dry up and now presents better appearance than it has at any time. Sach. lac.

4. Ibid. pp. 625-28.

July 7. Swollen gland became normal in few days, and in a month the lumps were so small they could scarcely be felt.

May 5 and June 4. Tuberculinum 50m was repeated. Had been having company and was very tired. Abscess at root of tooth, now. Glands swollen. Tuberc. cm.

Aug. 6. Instep—aching pain before menses, was reported two weeks after last report and has continued troublesome during and after walking. Tuberc. cm.

Aug. 31. Instep—aching continued in both feet so that she walked on the sides of the feet, when reported ten days ago. Has cold effects, now; Neck—a very sore spot, a lump too sore to be touched, slightly under the chin. Tuberc. cm. 4 powders; 1 each night and morning; Sach. lac. powders to follow, taken the same way.

Oct. 6. Swelling and suppuration of the old spot. So tired, constantly. Tuberc. mm.

Oct. 20. Feeling fine. Aching in insteps and soles returned.

Improvement continued throughout the year; the lumps disappeared from the neck and the pains disappeared from the feet. A cough in November was cured by Bry. 10m., and later the same month Tuberc. mm. was repeated.

In May and June, the system was weakened by overexertion which to some extent interfered with the action of the remedy. Hence it was repeated at closer intervals than would have been done, had the course of its action had no interruption.

In August, when the remedy was to be given in the cm. potency for the third time, four doses were administered in succession at twelve-hour intervals, to push the action of the remedy.

The progress of the case throughout is delightful, even to read. Without operation, the glands of tubercular nature disappeared from the neck and gouty pains appeared in the extremities. As these disappeared, the patient was cured of tuberculosis and of gouty tendencies simultaneously, and became a robust, hearty, stout, strong woman.[5]

People frequently ask whether homeopathy can cure cancer. Since contemporary diagnostic tools were not available in Kent's time, it is impossible to say whether the tumor in the following case was indeed malignant or not. In any event, since treatment is always directed toward the patient rather than toward a diagnostic category, an isolated case of

5. Ibid., pp. 633–34.

the cure of a tumor simply means that in this case the patient recovered.

This case also illustrates well the Victorian attitude toward women. Possibly one of homeopathy's attractions during Kent's time was that the homeopath could often prescribe on the basis of his own observations and the patient's verbal report, without having to subject the female patient to a thorough physical examination. Of course, with our more enlightened attitudes today, the physical examination is considered indispensable, in homeopathy as well as in allopathy.

June 1, 1888.—Miss A.W., aged thirty, Irish housemaid. Pelvic tumor, about which opinion varied. Abdomen resembled pregnancy of nine months. Her friends refused to go upon the street with her because of her appearance. She consulted several surgeons, and some declined to operate. The tumor could not be moved, seemed to fill the pelvic cavity. Its origin could not be traced; tumor was very hard. It being immovable, very hard and painful, were the reasons why one surgeon could not operate. No vaginal examination was made by me. She came to my office because she had heard that a local examination would not be made. She dates her discovery of it to five years ago. For two years she has felt much pain in the pelvis. Swelling of the pit of the stomach below the abdomen became distended. Feet oedematous. Constant headache; cold milk causes pain. Cannot take cold things; everything must be warm. Nausea and vomiting. Everything eaten makes her sick and causes vomiting, vomiting after every meal. Constipation, no desire for stool for many days. Always feels a constriction about the waist from pressure upwards of the tumor. Distension in stomach after eating so little. Menses regular, with cramping pain, has always relieved it by whiskey. Starts suddenly from a noise. Restless, and sleeps badly. Teeth decayed young; they are dark colored. She says she felt a lump in the right side as large as a child's head, which was the first she felt of it, about four years ago, it was then very hard. Pain in this lump in the side has been felt from time to time. Feet burn; must remove the shoes to cool them. She says feet feel like there was mustard on them. Lycop. cm.

July 23d.—Up to a few days ago she had no vomiting, and the pain is much better. She is again feeling worse. Lyc. mm.

August 2nd.—Called to see if medicine was expected to make her worse. S.L. (*Saccharum lactis*)

August 9th.—Called to say the aggravations had passed off and that she was much better.

September 25th.—Continued to improve up to a few days ago. Symptoms returning. Vomiting after eating and pain in the stomach. Lycop. mm.

October 28th.—Symptoms all passed away until a few days ago the pain came back in the pylorus, and again she received Lyc. mm.

November 27th.—No symptoms. S.L.

December 13th.—Reports no symptoms. S.L.

January 7th.—The tumor has diminished some. No bloating of feet. Can move the tumor and can discern that it belongs to the right side of the pelvis.

January 26th.—Symptoms returning. Lyc. mm.

February 16th.—She is growing smaller about the abdomen and gaining in flesh and color.

March 7th.—improving, No symptoms.

March 28th.—Still improving.

April 25th.—Stomach symptoms returning. Lyc. mm.

June 3rd.—Has been entirely free from symptoms until recently. Feet swelling again; cannot drink water nor cold milk; cannot take cold things; everything must be warm. Headache in forehead and eyes; pain in lumbar region; bowels constipated; now goes three or four days; feet burn. Lyc. mm.

June 15th.—Symptoms all better.

August 15th.—All symptoms have returned. She returns when the symptoms return. Lyc. 2 mm.

October 7th.—Reports herself cured. The tumor can be discovered by close examination. She had not been able to find it, therefore she thought she was cured. She remarked that the last medicine did her most good of all the medicine taken. She remains in perfect health.[6]

SOME MODERN CASES

How does homeopathy work in infectious diseases? The following acute case of gonorrhea, with laboratory smears confirming both the diagnosis and the cure, raises some provocative questions as to the necessity of treating venereal disease with the usual antibiotics. In recent times, Elizabeth Wright Hubbard was one of the prominent American proponents of strict Kentian prescribing.

6. Ibid., pp. 612–14.

CASE III. Woman, 40; one child; hysterectomy years ago; has sudden profuse thick yellow burning leuckorrhea, two days' duration, with bearing down sensation. Craving for sours since onset; all-gone sensation, nausea. Violent burning urination and frequency; pain up the rectum on urinating. Smear 4 plus for gonnorhea. *Sepia* 10M., one dose. Second smear on third day, 1 plus. Distress almost gone. Smears at one-week intervals all negative thereafter. Monthly checks since negative. General health better than in years.[7]

Homeopathy has been successful in treating diabetes over the years. The following study by Julia Green demonstrates that the dosage of insulin can be reduced; and sometimes insulin can be eliminated entirely. Because diabetes leads to organic changes, such as the destruction of nerve tissue, the patient in this case did lose some eyesight, which could not be restored.

CASE VI. Another case of my own.

L.E.M., medium height, stocky, rather pasty, sallow, very puffy about the eyes. In U.S. Naval Academy with rigid tests and O.K.

HISTORY: 1906: Trace of sugar in urine. 1908: Typhoid; never regained weight. 1911: Appendectomy; appendix found shrivelled; followed by abscess on abdominal wall. 1912: Some sugar but gradually less. 1914: Strangulated intestine, emergency operation. Sugar in quantity after this. One time of coma. 1916: Retired on account of diabetes. 1921: Gradual loss of weight. Neuralgia legs and feet until hard to walk. Began insulin; on it all the time since May, 1923.

HOMOEOPATHIC TREATMENT: June 16, 1925. Forty-two years, height 67¾ inches, weight 143½. At lowest weighed 113 and some of this oedema. Face sallow with tendency to moth spots and acne. B.P. below 100 at one time, now 130. Sugar in urine was 5 or 6%, now none for a year. Blood sugar was 35.00% two or three years ago, now none. Taking 32 units of insulin daily.

Left antrum has been infected for three years. Now slight discharge which is offensive. Skin extremely dry. Slight wounds or scratches very slow to heal. Ulcers over tibiae and between toes do not heal. Endurance low, must lie down frequently. Teeth poor, better since started insulin. Likes dry weather, mild climate. Worse damp weather and drafts. Craves open air. Calm naturally, phlegmatic, rather slow. Irritable with diabetes.

7. Elizabeth Wright Hubbard, M.D., "Nervous Moments of a 'G.P.',"
Homoeopathic Recorder 55, no. 11 (November 1940): 20.

July 14. Cut insulin one-half. *Lyc.* 10M. July 20. Decidedly better and cut out insulin. July 29. Stools regular (had been constipated many years). Diarrhoea the 24th. Aug. 10. Sugar 1⅛% a week ago.

Sept. 9. More energy; color better. Urinalysis ten days ago: quantity normal; sp. gr. 1036, sugar 2½%.

Oct. 24. More nervous, irritable. *Lyc.* 10M. Nov. 25. No better, very irritable. Sugar 3¾%. *Lyc.* 50M. Dec. 9. Better in general. Sugar 4%, sp. gr. 34.

Feb. 8, 1926. Growing worse, thinner, weaker. Vision blurred on attempting to read. Ulcer of great toe refuses to heal. *Sulph.* 10M.

Feb. 19. No better. Went to Naval Dispensary for examination. Advised return to insulin and did so. Told trouble with retina. *Psor.* 10M.

March 25. Gaining flesh steadily. Able to reduce quantity of insulin over and over and get a reaction, even when eating more freely than for years.

April 7. Urine and blood sugar free since early February. April 26. Has gained ten pounds. Looks more sallow. Eyes no better. *Psor.* 10M.

May 24. Insulin 18 units (one year ago 36 units). Vision better slowly. July 7. Vision worse. Ankles swelling. *Psor.* 50M.

Sept. 28. Able to go touring, driving long distances, eating as other people do in hotels and restaurants; careful to avoid most sweets.

Dec. 18. Been better. Now weight less. *Psor.* 50M.

Feb. 16, 1927. Toe which has had ulcer since treatment began entirely healed. Subsequent history is a repetition. Weight, strength, energy, remain good. Does all kinds of mechanical labor. Diet only slightly restricted. Insulin produces reaction occasionally and must be reduced. Vision is permanently affected so cannot read fine print. All tests for sugar negative.

The change from an invalid to a vigorous active man began promptly and has continued all these years; it would have to be seen to be realized. Remedies have been: *Psorinum* for a basic remedy; *Lycopodium* and *Sulphur* for lesser chronic ills and *Kali bi.* for acute troubles, mostly catarrhal.

The homoeopathic treatment for the diabetic is the same as for any other disorder and the results are very frequently soul satisfying.[8]

8. Julia M. Green, M.D., "The Effects of Homoeopathic Treatment on Diabetes," *Homoeopathic Recorder* 58, no. 3 (September 1941): 136–37.

Developmental problems in children often respond spectacularly to homeopathic prescribing. Elizabeth Wright Hubbard reports on a case of severe retardation that responded
to a series of remedies, including the nosode *medorrhinum*,
which was given on the basis of the mother's history of a
vaginal discharge. Note that when the child shows signs of
having contracted an acute disease—chicken pox—homeopathic treatment is directed at encouraging the symptoms
rather than suppressing them. Homeopaths teach that childhood diseases are valuable in that they confer important
immunity mechanisms on the patient and thus reduce susceptibility later in life.

Three months ago a young couple stepped tentatively into my
office. The wife looked like a 13th Century Madonna, thin and
worn, holding in her arms a little pallid, slanting-eyed boy of about
a year and a half. The father wept quietly as he told me that several
clinics and specialists had pronounced their little boy a Mongolian
idiot and had said that nothing could be done for him but custodial
care in some institution for his ilk. They had heard of Homoeopathy
and asked me if I thought anything at all could be done for the boy.

The child was thin and pasty-looking, his mouth open, drooling
slightly, with a sort of snorting snuffle every few breaths; his head
shape was within the limits of normal and his ears normal. He had
no teeth. He could neither stand nor sit without support, nor creep,
and his head would wobble if he got off balance. He was totally
unable to grasp anything. The mother said he could neither drink
from a cup nor suck at a bottle; she fed him with a spoon. When I
picked him up the musculature of his back and limbs was pitifully
flabby, like a rag doll. He seemed perfectly formed except for the
typical Mongoloid eye-casings. He did not smile or reach for bright
jewelry; he frequently put his head back and rolled his eyes toward
the ceiling and then flopped his head down on his chest. The
parents begged me not to give them any ray of hope, if there was
none. A more inexpressive and hopeless trio I have rarely seen.
The child had had no colds or childhood disease, no eruption,
convulsion, fright or accident.

What to do? All I could see was triple grief. I asked the mother to
tell me about her pregnancy and labour. She had experienced a
deep grief in the early months of her pregnancy, no nausea, easy
labour, no instruments needed. This was the second child, the elder
one being, they said, well and normal. No history of syphilis,

convulsions, or insanity in the family. Laboratory work under the previous doctors was all negative, including Wassermann, blood count, etc. The boy received one dose of *Natrum mur.* 10M on the tongue which he made no effort either to swallow or to spit. I explained to the parents what homoeopathic remedies can often do in sub-normal children and asked them to give me a try for at least three months, seeing the child every fortnight. I told them it might take several years to get much of anywhere.

Two weeks later, the child looked almost rosy and had a gleam of intelligence. The muscles of the back had better tone, he rolled his head and eyes less. He had begun to have a thick catarrh and almost a wheeze. The mother volunteered that he could now roll in bed and that he had taken to doing the queerest thing, sleeping with his little behind, as she called his buttocks, up in the air. The father was not present this time and I asked the mother if she had at any time had a sudden, creamy, profuse discharge from the womb. She said, "Why, yes, the year before this boy was born; but it was soon cleared up at the clinic." *Medorrhinum* 1M, one dose.

Two weeks later when I picked the baby up he grasped my hair. The snuffles and snorting were entirely gone, he had cut two teeth without trouble, could sit alone and was trying to pull himself up in his pen. He had a curious symptom of protruding the tongue between the lips and there was a gurgling sound when he drank. The mother told me he had been exposed to chicken pox and I found a few small spots on the abdomen. He had a short, concussive cough. I explained to her that it would do him good to have the chicken pox and have it thoroughly, but that he would need a remedy to help the vitality bring it well out, and gave him *Cuprum* 1M, one dose. He skipped the next visit because he blossomed out with a strong chicken pox rash. He himself seemed bright and better than he had ever been during the illness. When he returned at the end of a month he had gained three pounds, no longer stuck out his tongue, grasped my finger so tightly I could hardly extricate it and clutched the paper weight and pencils on my desk, and was beginning to make sounds such as "Dada" (he was by this time two years old). He felt far heavier than before, now had occipital head sweat with sour odor and was starting to cut two more teeth. *Calcarea carb.* 10M was given, on which he is still riding and gradually improving.

I have had occasion to do the mother's chronic case. Her remedy was *Sulphur.* I should judge the father's to be *Natrum mur.*

How far along toward normalcy will Homoeopathy be able to bring this child?[9]

9. Elizabeth Wright Hubbard, M.D., "The Run of the Mill," *Homoeo-pathic Recorder* 43, no. 8 (February 1948): 171–72.

Orthodox medicine has yet to find a cure for muscular dystrophy. In the following case, by treating the patient on the basis of her symptoms, Julia Green was able to produce a remarkable improvement in a girl with a complex miasmatic history.

Since cases of progressive muscular dystrophy are rare, it is interesting to have two in one long practice. The first was reported to the I.H.A. in the early 1930s; it is sketched again here for purposes of comparison.

M.C. was four and a half years old when I first saw her in March, 1931. Up to about that time she had seemed to her parents a healthy child but her inheritance was bad. On the paternal side a greatgrandmother had had tuberculosis, a grandmother cancer of the uterus, a grandfather died of spinal meningitis after hard drinking for many years. On the maternal side a greatgrandmother had had a paralytic stroke and a grandmother several strokes, an uncle died from a stroke, a great aunt had "leaky" heart valves, an aunt tuberculosis, an uncle paralysis from drinking jamaica ginger. The outlook from the point of view of heredity certainly was bad.

A year before I saw her, this child had been walking to her sister's school in the morning and again at noon, each way nine-tenths of a mile; making four miles five days a week. Also she took dancing lessons at that time.

At four and a half she was losing weight steadily, losing appetite, had increasingly poor color tending to be bluish in tint, was giving up play more and more to sit in on the sidelines, was developing fear of anything unusual. On physical examination hollows were noted where muscles ought to be, with a white nodular appearance of the skin over the hollow places. She would stumble and fall easily, would get down on her knees like an old person, would pull herself up with her arms, was very slow dressing and undressing. She had slight fever in spells.

I gave her *Sulph.* 10M in March and *Calc. c.* at the end of June. At that time her abdomen had become large and hard; she had noisy flatulence; her legs were looking like sticks. After the *Calc.*, vitality and appetite improved, but the atrophy was progressive. By July she was apt to fall prone and strike her forehead. By October she was pulling herself upstairs with her hands on the banisters or hands on knees. She could not get up off the floor alone, could not get into a chair, had to be lifted, but she took more interest in life and in other children.

In this month of October the parents decided to take her to Johns

Hopkins as the oracle of last resort. She stayed there in hospital for a week of observation and testing. Then the parents were given a letter signed by two heads of clinics stating the diagnosis, progressive muscular dystrophy, the prognosis, "no known cure," a few years to live, not beyond ten years of age probably, during which time she would become helpless and progressively weaker. So the despairing father and mother brought their child home and in a few days the father committed suicide because he could not face the future. This did not help matters any for the mother was left with two little children and a heavily mortgaged house.

I could think of only two remedies for this case, *Calc. c.* and *Phos.* I had her on one from June to November and on the other from November to January, 1932. Each one produced some improvement in strength, appetite and mental vigor, but neither produced a permanent gain or stopped the progress of the disease. By November it had become almost impossible for her to turn over in bed.

Then, on January 21st, I gave her *Calc. phos.* 10M and by February 17th, she looked decidedly better, had begun to gain weight. The muscles were really harder, more filled out, and she could handle herself slightly better.

From this time on changes for the better were steady and remarkable. In April she could run, picking feet up off the floor. In May she could walk and run normally. By August she could do almost anything other children could do, could go upstairs one foot over the other without holding the railing, could skip on one foot.

The next summer (1933) she was on a farm, climbing fences, excelling in games, called the tomboy of the group.

She has had no trouble with muscles since. She is tall, erect, wiry, with reddish hair and freckles. Tubercular inheritance showed for a time in frequent colds and coughs, also in enlarged lymphatics. Psoric tendencies were expressed in hay-fever for a few years in the spring and in eczema on back and limbs. Sycotic taint showed in large warts and huge callouses on one heel. Dysmenorrhea is present too.

She looks in blooming health, however. She has been an office worker the last few years and was happily married in April this year.[10]

Speech impediments present difficulties for orthodox medicine, and generally, the only specific treatment given is

10. Julia M. Green, M.D., "Two Cases of Progressive Muscular Dystrophy," *Homoeopathic Recorder* 64, no. 6 (December 1948): 139–40.

speech therapy. In the following case, a speech impediment of long standing is shown to respond to homeopathic medication.

Sept. 3., 1952. Large, stout, ruddy complexion, rather jolly female, single, 25 years old.

In early childhood began stammering; some of this ever since, greatly aggravated during the last year when mouth feels overfull of tongue.

Tongue large, heavy, in her way; wakes her from discomfort; any position, somewhat better lying prone. Numbness tongue marked. Much in the way when starts to talk; if talks on and on can do better. If stops liable to stammer badly.

Sensation as if region of tonsils too full of tissue, in the way (tonsils removed twice).

Sometimes can form the words but the sound will not come; sometimes lips tremble when word comes out.

Stammering: worse if excited; emotionally disturbed, etc. Blushes easily.

Head feels too heavy if sits in an audience long time; wants to hold up with her hands; this slightly worse left side. No headache.

Desire fresh air always. Likes all kinds of weather.

Tendency to colds from other people.

Appetite very large, likes everything. Little thirst.

Quick motioned.

In June severe attack prevalent epidemic with high fever for a week.

Worse air-conditioning; fan blowing; never in outdoor air. Rx *Belladonna* 2C.

Sept. 20: Can talk decidedly better; better when excited or emotionally upset any other way. Not so much pain or symptoms around mouth and chin, neck. Tongue not so much in the way. Sharp, stitching pains here and there over the body; come and go, remain for appreciable time but not long. Throat very sore on day after last medicine.

Sept. 26: Symptoms returning; even the speech worse again. Rx *Calc. c.* 10M.

Oct. 20: Voice remains worse, quite difficult to get the words out; then cannot keep talking as long until gets caught again. Inflamed throat right side with pain face, neck. New inflamed area hard palate. Rx *Calc. c.* 10M.

Oct. 31: Voice ever so much better; all around her remarking how much better she is. Bad as ever occasionally after hurrying or if very nervous.

Nov. 25. Going backward a bit in speech. Rx *Calc. c.* 10M.

Jan. 10, 1953: Chronic symptoms worse again with sore throat added and some cough. Speech decidedly worse again though can finish long sentences when gets over the initial stammering. Rx *Calc. c.* CM.

April 10: Last medicine worked like magic. Can talk almost like other people.[11]

In the following course of treating a severe case of epilepsy, Dr. Royal Hayes notes the progression of symptoms according to Hering's law, with symptoms appearing on the more external parts of the body as the problems with the nervous system subside.

A young married woman, with epilepsy gravior since appendectomy five years previous; frequent attacks, sometimes three in a day; delayed and painful menstruation, no morning appetite, faint stomach at 11 a.m. Pounding headaches every 8–9 days; weeping spells. Fincke's *Sulphur* 5M.

A month later, no headaches; hungry but too "full" to eat, cannot eat until 10 a.m. Urgent thirst for cold and craving for ice cream and sour things but aversion to sweets. *Phos.* 200th. Dunham's.

No attacks for a month then one. *Phos.* 200. No attacks for five months, then three. *Sulphur* 10M. Skinner's. No attacks during the last thirteen years. But she threw out boils, a rectal abscess, and had two attacks of psoriasis, meanwhile having *Sulphur* again, then *Calcarea.* Eczema then came out which was cured with *Nitric acid.*[12]

Although homeopathy does not claim to be able to cure terminal cases where tissue change is far advanced, it often effects remarkable changes in illnesses that have been given up by orthodox practitioners, as illustrated by Dr. Margery Blackie's following report of a case of nephrosis:

I want to mention one other group of cases and they are the hopeless cases.

A man came in to see me one day, to ask if I could see his wife in one of the big teaching hospitals, because she had been there for three months with a nephrosis. She had seen many famous urolo-

11. Julia M. Green, M.D., "Case Report," *Homoeopathic Recorder* 69, no. 10 (April 1954): 272–73.

12. Royal E. S. Hayes, M.D., "Miscellaneous Hits," *Homoeopathic Recorder* 45, no. 8 (August 1970): 591.

gists and they had pronounced that at most she had only a week to live now. He had asked that if that was the case then might she see a homoeopath. So I went and met the specialists on the spot and was given all the necessary information about her. She had had a very intensive course of prednisone for twelve weeks. She was swollen everywhere. Her blood urea was 180. I gave her *Eel serum* and in forty-eight hours her blood was down to 140 and the R.M.O. was delighted and thought she was going to live. However, when I next went in he was very gloomy and she was semi-comatose, very bluish in appearance and while I was there came-to suddenly and said, "Where is my letter, who has taken it? I don't want my things removed," and sunk again into semi-consciousness. So I gave her *Lachesis* and left a note for the specialist that it was one of the snake venoms and that Lord Horder had said that the only people who knew anything about snake venoms were the homoeopaths. In twenty-four hours she was a different person and went out in three weeks, very well. No one acknowledged that the homoeopathic remedies had done anything but when she had a very slight relapse two years later, I was sent for at once, and this time gave *Eel serum* 12 with a very good result.[13]

The following case illustrates the application of *arsenicum album* in an emergency case of food poisoning.

The first case, dating from July 1956, is an example of an acute emergency for which I was called to the house at 5 a.m. to find the patient, Miss J.L., age 22 years, in a state of collapse.

The history	was that of severe diarrhoea and nausea since 2:30 a.m. She had passed undigested food, also ½ pint of blood. The night before the whole family had partaken of a small meal at London Airport, the patient being the only one to suffer ill effects.
On examination	at 5 a.m. I found severe restlessness; the patient was collapsed and almost pulseless. She was dehydrated; the abdomen was scaphoid; and she was conscious and acutely anxious.

The clinical diagnosis was acute food poisoning.

13. Margery G. Blackie, "The Future of Homoeopathy," *British Homoeopathic Journal* 60, no. 1 (January 1971): 9.

<u>The treatment</u>	given was *Arsenicum album* 6. Three tablets were dissolved in water and the liquid trickled through the lips, at first every two minutes, then five, and continued at 15-minute intervals.
<u>Progress</u>	The pulse improved steadily, and the patient became more alert. By 6 a.m. she was still very weak but very much better. By 7:30 a.m. she was sitting up, and by 10 a.m. had eaten a small meal.
<u>The recovery</u>	was complete and uninterrupted.
<u>Pathological investigations</u>	Culture of stool sterile.[14]

Since orthodox medicine has no specific treatment for viral infections, serious cases of viral pneumonia can only be treated by oblique means. Antibiotics, although they cannot eradicate viral infections, are often given to prevent superinfection with bacterial organisms. In severe cases of pneumonia, if the situation is so urgent that there is no time to work out the proper homeopathic remedy, the homeopath might resort to antibiotics. In the following case, however, Dr. Dorothy Cooper was able to prescribe homeopathically and effect a remarkable recovery in an elderly patient.

My next two cases are examples of severe pneumonia, clearly demonstrating the advantage of homoeopathic over antibiotic treatment. The first case is that of a 73-year-old Scotsman, recently retired from service in India, to whom I was called on 26 June 1960. He had arrived from Oberammergau the previous night to stay with his niece, and thought he had thrown off a slight cold.

<u>History</u>	During the morning of the day on which I was called he had developed a fever, with temperature 102°–103° and had been awake all night with a hard cough. Sputum had been blood-stained on two occasions, with bright red streaks.

14. Dorothy J. Cooper, "Some Clinical Experiences," *British Homoeopathic Journal* 63, no. 2 (April 1974): 102.

He was normally tough and threw off colds, but this time he felt ill.

On examination

At 7:30 p.m., I found him to be a silent man. His temperature was 102°. Pulse 90. Respiration 24. He had a hard, dry, irritating cough. He held his wife's hand and seemed afraid to be left alone.
His throat and nares were acutely inflamed. Examination of the chest revealed percussion note dull at the left base, with patchy bronchovesicular breathing. There were fine crepitations left apex anteriorly.

Clinical diagnosis

Virus pneumonia involving left apex and left base.

Treatment

He was given *Phosphorus* 1M 2-hourly for 48 hours.

Pathological Report Summary

"Sedimentation rate maximal all methods. The whole picture is quite consistent with virus pneumonia."

Progress

The following day he was very much better, with a temperature of 98°.
Pulse 80. Respiration 18.
His cough was less severe and he had been able to sleep.
Chest examination revealed fine crepitations left base, otherwise physical signs had not changed. Next day he reported having slept well, undisturbed by coughing.
Temperature remained 98°.
Pulse was down to 76.
Respiration was 16.
Chest: left apex clear, left base prolonged expiratory sounds but no crepitations.
He then told me he always had an 8-day fever with any cold, with a maximal rise at 4–8 p.m., then dropping. This had never been accounted for by blood examination.

Treatment

Lycopodium 1M 2-hourly was given.

Progress

On 29 June 1960, i.e. the third day, the temperature remained normal and the patient was in excellent form.

Chest: showed no abnormal physical signs apex or base. So on that day I gave permission for him to return home to Scotland two days later.

Two extracts from subsequent letters complete the history. On 10 July he wrote "My own doctor thinks I have been lucky", and 14 July, "am pretty well on my feet again, thanks to your drastic remedies!" (a non-homoeopathic patient).

Comment

To me the most notable points here are his rapid response to the *Phosphorus* followed by *Lycopodium* so that only 72 hours after the onset, the patient was not only fit to travel to Scotland by car, but all abnormal physical signs in his chest had cleared.[15]

An undescended testicle in a twelve year old would have to be treated surgically by orthodox medicine, and it might not be curable. The rapid response after administration of the homeopathic remedy in this case cannot be attributed to "spontaneous remission." It is unfortunate that Dr. Pratt does not document the symptoms upon which he prescribed.

A boy, aged 12, had his left testis normally descended but his right testis was in the inguinal canal. Operation had been advised. *Aurum met.* 30, 3 doses, was prescribed; 9 days later his mother phoned to say that the testis was now in the scrotum all the time. Follow-up, 1 year later, showed that the descent was permanent.[16]

In the following case, Dr. Roger Schmidt underlines the importance of educating the patient about the direction of cure. Since the history starts with recurrent skin eruptions that were repeatedly suppressed, Dr. Schmidt warns the patient not to interfere with the action of the remedy as the symptoms are once again brought to the surface and to the extremities.

Mr. G.B., 72 years old, told me he suffered, when he was about 40, from an obdurate eczema which had extended from the feet to

15. Ibid., pp. 102–104.

16. N. J. Pratt, "Homoeopathic Case Review," *British Homoeopathic Journal* 63, no. 1 (January 1974): 15.

the sexual parts, then onto the trunk and at last to the eyelids and scalp. But for the eczema, he thought at that time that he was very strong and in perfect health. It required years of various treatment, and the use of numerous ointments to suppress little by little this eruption, traces of which are still to be seen on the scalp and eyelids. During more than twenty years since the time he had at last succeeded in ridding himself of his eczema, he suffered from frequent influenza, then from bronchitis, which little by little turned into asthma. He attributes all these phenomena, from which he never suffered before, to chills and these grew worse in spite of every care. Little by little rheumatism set in which made him suffer cruelly, in the shoulders, hands, and lower limbs. Every winter he had one or two attacks of lumbago and sciatica, without mentioning attacks of bronchitis and asthma.

Now he has a pityriasic erythema on the scalp, dry eczema of the eyelids and conjunctivitis. The skin all over the body is extremely dry and covered with little white scales, especially abundant on the limbs. When auscultating the globulous thorax one hears big rhonci and numerous sibilances spread about. The cough is noisy, paroxysmal, turns loose and dry. Solar plexus painful when pressed, when the patient is standing (signal pain according to Leven) which denotes a gastric ptosis. The liver, very sensitive to touch, continues beyond the ribs a little. The patient complains of lack of appetite and constipation. Dry arthritis of the shoulders and knees. Heart normal. Pulse 75. Arterial pressure 150/90. Tendon reflexes not very much marked. Numerous nodosities around the articulations of both hands. The nails of the big toes are very much thickened. The patient is frequently disturbed in his sleep by his cough and after 5 in the morning he cannot sleep at all.

This story and the complex of the present symptoms clearly indicate *Sulphur*. On January 27 I give *Sulphur* 30 every morning in the plus method. On February 3 the patient returns saying: "I feel better, I sleep better, till 6:30. The cough disappeared two days ago, the breathing is deeper, the stairs much less difficult to ascend. I have an appetite again, my bowels evacuate two or three times a day." The only shadow in the picture is the increase of "rheumatism" nearly everywhere. I give *Placebo*.

On February 27, the above mentioned improvements are maintained. The head is lighter, the mind more active, the ideas clearer. The itching and the erythema of the scalp have disappeared. The eyes are getting better. On the contrary, the rheumatic pains are stronger in the hands and feet. "An extraordinary thing, doctor, my previous perspirations and my eczema of 20 years ago, on the

genital parts, on the hands and feet have returned. I don't want to recommence that comedy of yore." I warn my patient and tell him to abstain from any external medicinal application and I speak to him of the law of cure explaining to him that his symptoms are following exactly the desired direction:
From above downward (the head is better, the lower parts of the body worse).
From within outward (the cough, asthma, breathing, digestive functions are very much improved, whilst the extremities show serious aggravation).
And in the reverse order of the coming of the symptoms (reappearance of the previous eczema and perspiration). Of course I give *Placebo*.

On April 2, I see my patient again. He declares that his state has rapidly improved, until a recent journey during which he indulged in an indiscretion of diet, which brought about a strong aggravation of all skin symptoms. The rheumatism is better but has not completely disappeared. I order a dose of *Sulphur* 200 and *Placebo*. (The duration of *Sulphur* 30 was 10 weeks.)

On July 6 the patient returns to thank me. He is cured and wishes to make me endorse his opinion. [17]

Homeopaths have reported great success in treating acne, that bane of adolescence. The following case of several years' standing is reported to improve in two weeks under treatment with the indicated homeopathic remedy.

Every week our consulting room is visited by doctors who are anxious to learn about homoeopathy. At a morning session when four doctors were present, we saw an eighteen year old girl suffering from the worse possible outbreak of acne. She gave us her background. Her parents had been separated and the skin trouble started four years ago after her mother's death and her father did not want her back. In fact nobody wanted her. An uncle said he would pay to equip her for a job but again she felt that he would want to be finished with her. She told us she was worried about her future and that her moods varied from hour to hour and that she was extremely constipated. *Natrum muriaticum* was prescribed in high potency and she was told to come back in a fortnight. When she did so one barely recognized the pretty bright girl who walked in with her face practically clear—she was only seen once more, but

17. Roger Schmidt, M.D., "The Law of Cure," *Homeotherapy* 1, no. 5 (1975): 13–14.

after a year she sent a request for more medicine. Her skin had been perfectly all right but she had been very worried over her first job, and she thought it might start again although it had not so far![18]

INTERVIEW WITH A PATIENT

What is homeopathic treatment like from the patient's point of view? The following interview with a patient of a homeopathic physician in California has been transcribed verbatim. At the time she began treatment, the patient knew nothing about homeopathy, and because of her mental state the doctor's explanations largely went unheeded. She has since begun to study the homeopathic philosophy, and as the interview illustrates, she now has some understanding of the homeopathic aggravation and the direction of cure in her own case.

A.D. is in her thirties, the mother of a son, aged eleven, and a daughter, aged eight. She is presently a student; she has worked in the past in medical offices.

Q: You said you were a patient of Dr. ———. When did you start going to him?

A: About two years ago.

Q: Why did you decide to go to him?

A: I had a nervous breakdown, sort of, after the separation from my husband, a total physical, mental—I was a mess. I developed asthma, and I had no energy, and I was drinking a lot. And it's funny, I went to the store to buy a six-pack of beer, and the clerk there—I was always friendly with him—he started talking to me; he said, I know who you should see. He had never seen him, but he knew of somebody who had. And I called up and made an appointment; I didn't know what homeopathy was.

Q: Had you thought about going to any other kind of doctor before that?

A: I had been. I'd been going to an internist.

Q: And this was for treatment of the asthma?

18. Margery G. Blackie, *The Patient, Not the Cure* (London: Macdonald and Jane's, 1976), pp. 109–110.

A: Asthma and nerves. Because I would hyperventilate and pass out. I couldn't go into restaurants. I had to have a friend do my grocery shopping for me. I could make it to the store to pick up a six-pack and that was it. This had never happened to me in my whole life.

Q: How long was this going on?

A: It was going on for about six months. And the internist had me on an asthma medication plus eighty milligrams of Librium a day. And I was zonked. The Tedral for the asthma makes you hyper, nervous, and then the Librium of course made me just like this ["zonked" expression], and I was depressed.

Q: In other words, you weren't feeling any real effects from the treatment you were getting; it wasn't making you any better.

A: I was getting worse. Because the asthma has to do with the nerves. So that if you're taking medication that makes you more nervous, it doesn't work. Anyway, the internist knew he couldn't help me. He sent me to a psychiatrist. I was going to a psychiatrist once a week—that cost me fifty dollars a week—with no results.

Q: The psychiatrist wasn't giving you any separate medi cations?

A: No, he knew I was on Librium. It's the strangest thing—I mean, I just can't explain what was going on at that time. I don't know if you know what it feels like to not have one bit of energy, not be able to breathe. And everybody, I think, has that at certain times in their lives for maybe a short time, but this was just going on and on. It was scary. So, as soon as I started going to Dr. ———, I didn't take any drugs. I immediately got off the drugs, and it was tough because he immediately put me on a fast, too, to clear my system of the drugs—a juice fast, for seven days. And he gave me a remedy that put me in bed for three days with the worst asthma attack I've ever had.

Q: Do you know what the remedy was?

A: Sulfur.

Q: Did he give it to you right away, while you were fasting, or after you finished the fast?

A: He gave it to me immediately.

Q: And you were in bed for three days?

A: Yeah, I just could not move. I was so sick.

Q: How had your asthma been up to that time? I'm just trying to get an idea of whether this was a result of discontinuing the drugs or whether it was an aggravation.

A: It was an aggravation. I mean, my asthma was bad, but it wasn't to the point where I couldn't get out of bed.

Q: Had he warned you that this would happen?

A: Yeah. He *hoped* it would happen.

Q: Did he explain what homeopathic treatment involved before he gave you anything?

A: He did, but as I say, I was zonked. I went in there— and I'm a very assertive person, and people don't manipulate me, but what I wanted was to be put away, and I kept trying to convince my psychiatrist to put me away, and so I didn't care. All I knew was I couldn't carry on. The kids took care of me, it was the strangest thing. But as soon as I went through that remedy, that three days, I was a different human being.

Q: What kinds of changes did you see?

A: My lungs immediately cleared up; I had always had a lot of wheezing and stuff. And as I remember, I immediately enrolled back in school, and I started dating.

Q: This was immediately after you got out of bed.

A: Immediately! I mean, the improvement— But since then, see, I have apparently antidoted myself in some way. And the symptoms have changed. The way I understand it in homeopathy, it's like opening a can of worms. That was just one layer. I immediately felt an improvement, but there were other things, and so we've been trying to work with it ever since. And I've had setbacks and I've gone down.

Q: Have you ever been as bad as when you started?

A: Never.

Q: So it's always been a gradual improvement. Have you had changes of remedy over time?

A: Lots of different remedies.

Q: Have you seen any evidence of the symptoms going in the direction of Hering's law?

A: I don't know what that is.

Q; Well, according to Hering, when you're under constitutional treatment with homeopathic remedies, your symptoms disappear in a definite order, and the innermost part of you is what recovers first, and then you start developing symptoms more outward. Did you notice anything like that?

A: Immediately after most of the remedies I've had, especially the last remedy, which was *Lycopodium*, I went into a very deep emotional depression, and suicidal feelings. This was three days after taking the remedy. And I've had it off and on with other things too, but usually there's that emotional reaction. And then I've had, oh, skin rashes and—

Q: How soon after taking the remedy have those appeared?

A: I've taken so many, it's really hard to remember. If you want to talk about the last one, maybe that would be best for me. Right after he gave me the *Lycopodium*, I had a lot of energy. Three days later I was in total depression. And that lasted for a couple days, and then I became extremely anxious. But it wasn't as deep as what I'd felt before, because I knew in the back of my head that I was going to be over it. And I started calling people, calling my friends, calling the Wholistic Health Center and talking to the secretary—you know, I knew it was going to pass but I didn't know when. And that lasted about two weeks. But then, after that, I had kidney symptoms.

Q: Had you ever had those before?

A: Yeah, I used to have a lot of kidney problems.

Q: How long ago?

A: I think about three years ago now. But I had them for years and years; I had them for eight years, but three years ago was the last really bad episode. Kidney stones.

Q: You had kidney stones?

A: Millions. But I haven't had them since I've been going to Dr. ———.

Q: So the kidney symptoms you had were less severe than the actual presence of stones.

A: Oh, yeah, I never actually had an infection or bleeding with this last episode; it just lasted for a few hours of pain.

Q: Just pain but no visible symptoms?

A: No. And then I got athlete's foot, which was very strange.

Q: This was on *Lycopodium?*

A: Yes. And I had a vaginal infection that lasted a whole week.

Q: Was that an old symptom too, or was this the first time?

A: I had had one before, a couple of years ago, which was a yeast infection. But, see, I never had this checked out to see what it was because I knew it was part of the remedy.

Q: Had the yeast infection previously been treated with medication?

A: Antibiotics. But this just went away within a week. It wasn't nearly as bad as the yeast infection that I had, but it was uncomfortable.

Q: Have you had any acute diseases while you've been under treatment, like any infectious diseases, flu, anything like that?

A: I've had the flu a couple of times.

Q: Did you get treated for that separately?

A: No, I didn't get treated. I think that's one of the things that's changed in me so much. I don't treat things anymore, I just suffer through them.

Q: Did you notice any difference in the way you reacted to the flu, from when you had it before?

A: It was much shorter. I noticed that. One was a stomach flu, where it was just severe vomiting for five or six hours, and then two days later I was fine. Things don't hang on anymore. I don't seem to have any more allergies to things.

Q: You said that you were drinking a lot at the time you went to Dr. ———. Did that just stop by itself, or were you making an effort to cut down on drinking, or are you still drinking a lot?

A: I go through these phases of cutting down. I still drink a lot, but nothing like I did. I don't drink to get drunk; I just don't get drunk. Because I used to try to blot myself out. But I still seem to need those three or four beers, or three or four glasses of wine, at night. But it's a whole different attitude about drinking.

Q: What is your feeling in general about the way you're relating to your body, the way that you're reacting to disease? Do you feel that you have more control over what's going on, that you have more consciousness of it?

A: I'll tell you, an episode happened right after my husband left. I woke up in the morning and my face and lips were swollen about five times their size. I'd been bitten by a spider and had an allergic reaction, which I've always had to bugs. And I went to the emergency hospital and they gave me some sort of antihistamine. And one doctor told me I should carry Adrenalin with me all the time, and another doctor told me that it's like waiting for a truck to hit me. And I was just so confused. I could not sleep for months. I was afraid of everything. I was just totally afraid that I was going to go to sleep, a spider was going to bite me, and I was going to die.

Q: This was during the period when you were having other really severe mental symptoms too?

A: Yeah, it was before Dr. ———. I would spray the room with bug killer. I was afraid to go in the woods. I was a nervous wreck. I'd have to drink to go to sleep. It was awful. I don't spray my room now. There's gobs of bugs around; you know, when you live in the woods there's a lot of them.

Q: And you're not getting a reaction to them?

A: No. I'm just not afraid anymore.

Q: Have you used any allopathic drugs at all since you started homeopathic treatment?

A: Let's see—now, that yeast infection, I did take something, that was the only thing. But I didn't know that that was a normal thing to happen.

Q: Dr. ——— was away during part of the time that you were under treatment. Did you communicate with him by mail?

A: Well, yes. P—— [another homeopath] communicated for me. She took all the data and sent it off, and she's the one who prescribed the *Lycopodium*. But see, I haven't had any problems. I didn't have any problems for a long, long time. Except just before I had this last bout of depression, I went in to have endodontics done on my teeth, and apparently that must have antidoted the remedy. And I had no idea that would happen. So I'm real careful, as much as I'd love to have a cup of coffee.

Q: You don't drink coffee anymore?

A: No. I used to drink a pot a day. I was just a fanatic for coffee. And now I drink decaffeinated coffee, and I'm pretty used to it, but real coffee sure smells good.

Q: What other remedies have you taken, can you remember?

A: *Pulsatilla*—and one time he gave me one that was off a little bit, and I broke out in a fungus all over. It was awful. But it went away quickly. That's the thing. It never seemed important to me because I wasn't interested in it as a science, so I didn't pay attention to what remedies I got. And I still don't really understand it. I'm learning more and more about it, but it's not that I understand *homeopathy*, it's that I understand health more.

PART III

HISTORICAL HOMEOPATHY

8

THE HISTORY OF HOMEOPATHY

In 1900, there were an estimated 15,000 homeopathic physicians practicing in the United States—about one-sixth of the medical profession. In 1976, the National Center for Homoeopathy, a branch of the only remaining national homeopathic organization in the United States, listed only about 225 physicians in its directory.

In 1900, homeopathy was a separate medical system, with its own schools and relatively active organizations and journals. Today homeopathy is formally classified as a subspecialty of internal medicine and is thus subsumed under the umbrella of allopathic practice. No homeopathic medical schools survive in this country; membership in the American Institute of Homeopathy (AIH), the only national homeopathic organization, has declined; and the homeopathic journals have dwindled to a handful.

Even though numbers of people are exploring homeopathy as an alternative to traditional medicine, its practice has contracted to the point that homeopathic treatment is unavailable in most communities of the United States.

The complex social, economic, and intellectual factors that caused such a decline cannot be completely delineated, but a brief review of the history of homeopathy will show that the decline was not principally due to any failure in actual medical practice.

HAHNEMANN'S REBELLION AGAINST ALLOPATHY

At the peak of its popularity, around the turn of the twentieth century, homeopathy was practiced in a wide variety of ways—ranging from strict adherence to Hahnemann's principles, to borrowings from the homeopathic pharmacopoeia by orthodox physicians, to the practice of homeopathy in the home with the assistance of manuals and prepared kits of remedies. However, when we speak of homeopathy in the United States today, we are referring to the doctrine formulated by Hahnemann and elaborated by those of his followers who placed the strictest interpretation upon the early homeopathic writings. To the contemporary practitioner of homeopathy, the practice of this healing art is as closely allied with the thought and personality of its founder as it was at the outset.

As might be expected, homeopathic advocates write of Hahnemann with near reverence, whereas biographical material from the mainstream of medical history tends to view him with a mixture of ridicule and pity for what orthodoxy considers his deluded insistence on a web of fanciful principles. Because writers about Hahnemann are generally approaching their subject from one camp or the other, it is difficult to gain a balanced view of the man. In the context of the state of the medical art of his time, however, we can understand what prompted Hahnemann's search for a new principle of therapeutics, and in that light we can better appreciate the significance of his contribution to medical thought.

Hahnemann formulated the principles of homeopathy around the beginning of the nineteenth century, a period during which every sphere of human activity was in a state of upheaval and disorder. The French Revolution and the national and international wars that followed it disrupted virtually every corner of Europe. The revolutionary spirit in France had brought a new emphasis on the value and dignity of the individual, a concept that was to play a large part in Hahnemann's thinking.

Despite the continually shifting theoretical ground of medicine in Hahnemann's time, regular medical practitioners generally resorted to the methods of "heroic" medicine: bloodletting, cupping, blistering, purging, sweating, and other strenuous and often fatal measures. In an effort to draw off what they considered to be excess blood, physicians would open a patient's veins and remove anywhere from several ounces to several quarts of blood. Leeches were sold in huge quantities for the same purpose. Hot cups were applied to a patient's skin, and as they cooled, a vacuum would be created, drawing blood to the surface. Harsh substances were placed or burned on the skin, and when the resulting second-degree burn became infected, the pus that exuded was taken as evidence that the infection was being drawn out of the body. Large doses of drugs were given to induce vomiting, to evacuate the bowels, and to produce sweating. In addition to these measures, large doses of calomel, or mercurous chloride, were administered, either as a specific in certain diseases or for mercury's ability to promote sweating and salivation. Strangely enough, the dangers of mercury poisoning were not unknown to the physicians of Hahnemann's time: loosening of teeth, deterioration of bones, and loss of hair were recognized as side effects of mercury treatment.

Not even the wealthiest and most powerful figures, with the best medical care available to them, were exempt from the dangers of such treatment. George Washington died following a sore throat and breathing difficulties, probably due as much to the heroic treatment he received as to his actual illness: during the afternoon and evening of the last day of his life, he was bled three times, having had at least four pints of blood removed, treated with blistering, and dosed with calomel.

Because Hahnemann gained much of his livelihood from the translation and annotation of scientific texts, he was conversant with developments in the "hard" sciences of his day. It is therefore even more remarkable that, unlike his medical colleagues, he did not hasten to adopt an isolated chemical or physical principle as the sole explanation of the origin and treatment of diseases. Rather, very much in the tradition of the experimental scientists, Hahnemann founded his doctrine of homeopathy on empirical evidence of the action of drugs. It was in his development of a set of principles according to which medicinal substances were to be used to treat disease that Hahnemann made his great contribution to medical thought. Even today, the very idea that there might be a unitary principle for the selection of medicines remains a revolutionary notion.

Hahnemann spent his early years in a bitter struggle to advance his scholarly pursuits. Born in 1755 in Meissen, in the Electorate of Saxony, Samuel Hahnemann knew a childhood of poverty. Although Samuel's father, a porcelain painter, fostered the boy's early interest in careful and difficult study, he removed the boy from school on several occasions in the hope of turning Samuel's interests toward a more rewarding occupation. When Samuel was taken out of school and sent to work for a greengrocer in Leipzig, the boy ran away and returned home, where his mother had to hide him for several days to protect him from the wrath of his father.

With the aid of a teacher who recognized Samuel's promise as a scholar, the boy was permitted to return to the local Latin school free of tuition. He was particularly gifted in languages; and at the age of twelve he reportedly assisted younger students with their beginning lessons in Greek. Hahnemann's eventual mastery of French, English, Italian, Greek, Hebrew, Arabic, and other languages was later to be put to good use when he turned to translating as a means of gaining a livelihood. His linguistic gifts also exposed him to much obscure medical and scientific literature that helped to reinforce his convictions about the universality of the doctrine he developed.

In 1775, Hahnemann left Meissen for Leipzig, where he began his study of medicine, supporting himself by tutoring in languages and doing translations. Because there was no hospital in Leipzig, he eventually left for Vienna, where he gained clinical experience as a protégé of the renowned Dr. Joseph von Quarin at the Brothers of Mercy Hospital. Hahnemann's funds soon ran out, and he finally accepted employment with the governor of Transylvania at Hermannstadt. In addition to cataloging the governor's library and classifying his coin collection, Hahnemann served as the governor's medical adviser and began practicing in the town, despite the fact that he had not yet qualified as a doctor—an indication of the lax professional standards of the day.

Finally, in 1779, at the age of twenty-four, Hahnemann had enough money to enroll at Erlangen, where he received his medical degree that same year. He set up his first practice in the copper-mining town of Hettstedt, but in 1781 he moved to Dessau, and the following year he married Henriette, the daughter of the local apothecary. Meanwhile he continued his studies in chemistry and other scientific fields, supplementing his earnings by doing translations.

The ensuing years were a time of crisis for Hahnemann. He and his growing family moved from town to town, changing their place of residence seventeen times over the next twenty years and always living in virtual poverty. Owing to his translations and annotations of major scientific works, Hahnemann began to acquire a reputation as a scholar and scientist. He also began to publish original works on public health issues and to openly criticize the dangerous medical practices of the day.

Increasingly disillusioned with the medical doctrines he had learned, and apprehensive of the harm done by the prevailing school, Hahnemann withdrew from the practice of medicine and devoted himself to chemical research, translation, and writing. Caught between the need to support his family and his mistrust of the medicine he had been taught, he had serious misgivings about practicing at all.

The turning point in Hahnemann's career came in 1790, while he was translating William Cullen's *Treatise of the Materia Medica*, an important work by a leading Scottish medical authority. In a section devoted to a discussion of Peruvian bark, also known as cinchona, the source of our modern quinine, Cullen attributed the bark's curative effect in intermittent fever (i.e., malaria) to its bitter and astringent qualities.

Hahnemann questioned this analysis and subsequently ingested the drug himself, an unusual experiment for an eighteenth-century physician, but not entirely without precedent. In 1789, Hahnemann had published a treatise on syphilis and gonorrhea which showed the influence of the Scottish physician, John Hunter. Hunter, in an attempt to gain firsthand knowledge of the development of syphilis in the infected individual, had inoculated himself with syphilitic material. Hunter's observation that the organism cannot be diseased in two ways simultaneously, and his idea that mercurial medicines (the cure for syphilis at the time) act to introduce a new, artificial irritation that displaces the initial irritation from the syphilitic poison, were undoubtedly forerunners of Hahnemann's homeopathic doctrine. Hahnemann, in his 1796 "Essay on a New Principle for Ascertaining the Curative Powers of Drugs, with a Few Glances at Those Hitherto Employed," introduced the two principles upon which homeopathy was to be founded. His experience in the cinchona experiment had convinced him that the curative power of the bark lay in its similarity to the disease it cured.

In the same essay, Hahnemann advocated the use of "provings" (from the German *Pruefung*—"test" or "trial") to determine the therapeutic powers of medicine. A remedy was to be given to healthy individuals, and all the symptoms they exhibited were to be recorded. The sick patient was then to be treated by administering the remedy whose symptom pattern from its provings was most similar to the symptoms of the illness.

Following the publication of the essay, Hahnemann returned to the practice of medicine, but now he began treating patients on the basis of the Law of Similars. In 1805, he established a practice in Torgau, and in that year he published a small volume of provings of twenty-seven medicines he had tested on himself.

In 1810 Hahnemann published the first edition of the *Organon of Rational Healing* (later retitled the *Organon of the Healing Art*), which systematically spelled out the principles of the homeopathic doctrine. The frank denunciation of orthodox medicine in the *Organon* intensified opposition to Hahnemann within the medical profession.

The *Organon* was not as successful as Hahnemann had hoped it would be in converting his colleagues to the new system, so in 1812 he moved to Leipzig and applied for permission to teach at the university. In order to qualify for the faculty, he was required to deliver a lecture, and he presented his historical study of the ancient use of white hellebore (*Veratrum album*) to a packed hall. It is testimony to the spreading curiosity about Hahnemann's revolutionary doctrine that doctors had come from far and near to hear his first public lecture. Although Hahnemann was already a controversial figure, his thesis, which avoided reference to the homeopathic doctrine, was accepted without opposition.

Hahnemann's course of lectures at the University of Leipzig was not particularly successful. The zeal with which he advocated absolute adherence to his new system, at the same time heaping scorn upon the practices of orthodox medicine, alienated many students, and attendance dropped steadily. Hahnemann and his faithful pupils also began to feel the antagonism of the regular medical profession within the university.

During this period Hahnemann began to gather around him a circle of followers—at first, medical students, and later, physicians and lay enthusiasts as well—who gathered at his home and performed provings of medicines under his direction. In 1811 and 1812 Hahnemann's *Materia Medica Pura* was published in six volumes, recording the extensive remedy provings that had been carried out by Hahnemann and his followers.

Despite the growing opposition to homeopathy among the ranks of orthodoxy, the new system scored a victory when it met with success in treating a typhus epidemic that was carried into Europe by Napoleon's army as they retreated from Moscow in 1813. With the impetus provided by such clinical successes, homeopathy began to spreading throughout Europe.

In addition to the attacks launched against Hahnemann within the medical profession, opposition was opened on another front by the apothecaries of Leipzig, who brought Hahnemann to court with the accusation that he was infringing on their privileges. In violation of a law requiring that all medicines be compounded and dispensed by pharmacists, Hahnemann had been preparing his own remedies and dispensing them to his patients. Hahnemann justifiably felt that the apothecaries would not be meticulous enough in preparing homeopathic remedies, and under the pressure of the apothecaries, he left Leipzig, and moved in 1821 to Anhalt-Koethen, accepting the invitation of Duke Ferdinand, to whom he became personal physician and who permitted him to prepare and dispense his own remedies. There, Hahnemann was able to pursue his practice in relative peace for the next fourteen years.

In 1828, after more than a decade of intense study, Hahnemann published his *Chronic Diseases*. This work drew new criticism from the orthodox medical profession, and Hahnemann's insistence that seven-eighths of man's ills could be traced to "psora"—generally understood as "the itch" (scabies)—created a rift within the growing ranks of homeopaths as well.

By 1829 homeopathy had achieved considerable stature, and when Hahnemann's medical golden jubilee was celebrated that year, he received visits and congratulations from prominent physicians and enthusiasts from all over Europe and abroad. Hahnemann's wife, Henriette, died six months later, and Hahnemann lived on in virtual isolation.

The new school of medicine had a chance to prove its effectiveness in 1831 and 1832 when an epidemic of Asiatic cholera swept into Europe. Thanks to a great-nephew who wrote him from Prague describing in minute detail the symptoms of the cholera victims in that city, Hahnemann was able to prescribe a series of remedies even before he had seen a single case of the dread disease. Wherever homeopathic remedies were used, significant reductions in the mortality rate were demonstrated. Part of the success of the homeopathic treatment lay in its gentle approach, as opposed to the harmful measures taken by orthodox physicians; nevertheless, even staunch adherents to orthodoxy began to use the remedies recommended by Hahnemann during the epidemic.

In 1834 a visitor appeared at Hahnemann's home. A young well-born Frenchwoman, Melanie d'Hervilly, arrived in town disguised as a boy and presented herself to Hahnemann, saying that she wanted to study homeopathy. In a short time Hahnemann and the young woman, who was less than half his age, were married, and she soon persuaded him to move to Paris. Homeopathy was well established in Paris by that time, and Hahnemann's arrival was greeted with rejoicing. During his last days Hahnemann enjoyed a busy practice among the elite of Paris society, and he was able to make use of his position in the intellectual center of Europe to popularize the homeopathic doctrine. He died in 1843 at the age of eighty-eight, and he was buried under rather peculiar circumstances: Melanie made no public announcement of his death, and his body was interred almost in secret in a small cemetery in Montmartre. Hahnemann's sixth edition of the *Organon* remained in Melanie's hands, and it was with considerable difficulty that the document finally became available for publication in the twentieth century. Largely through the efforts of American homeopaths, Hahnemann was reburied in Père Lachese in 1898, in the company of the immortals of France, and his tomb was finally allowed to bear the inscription he had requested: *Non inutilis vixi* ("I have not lived in vain").

Critics of Hahnemann have seized on his faults as justifications for their rejection of homeopathy, but such faults as he had were not particularly relevant to the truth of the homeopathic doctrine. He committed a serious scientific error when he announced the discovery of a new chemical compound, which on analysis turned out to be simple borax. Hahnemann acknowledged the mistake and published a detailed description of the procedure he had used that had led him to make his error. On another occasion, Hahnemann foolishly advertised a "secret remedy" that could be purchased for a certain fee. The secret turned out to be the use of *Belladonna* for scarlet fever. The remedy was indeed valuable, but Hahnemann's method of advertising it proved an embarrassment to the homeopathic cause.

Hahnemann's quick temper and his intolerance of the slightest deviation from his doctrine divided the ranks of his followers, and his invective against the practices of the orthodox profession did little to win converts to homeopathy. Had his zeal been tempered with tact, perhaps homeopathy might have been able to make more rapid inroads against the life-threatening forms of treatment that have continued to be used in allopathic practice long after Hahnemann's death.

HISTORY OF HOMEOPATHY IN THE UNITED STATES[1]

Introduction and Spread of Homeopathy

The first homeopathic physician in the United States was Dr. Hans Burch Gram, a Bostonian of Dutch extraction who received his medical education in Copenhagen, where he converted to the New School of homeopathy. When he returned to New York in 1825, he set up an exclusively homeopathic practice that became the focus for the spread of the doctrine through New York and the New England states, where the ranks of homeopathy were increased by converts from allopathy.

A Swiss-German physician, Dr. Henry Detwiller, came to Pennsylvania from Europe in 1817 and, after studying the doctrine through readings and correspondence, converted to the New School in 1828. A few years thereafter, Constantine Hering also settled in Pennsylvania, and through the influence of these two German homeopaths the doctrine spread throughout the German-speaking immigrant community.

In 1835, Detwiller and Hering established the first homeopathic academy in America in Allentown, Pennsylvania. All instruction was in German, and for this reason and others, the school was forced to close in 1841. In 1848, in Philadelphia, Hering established the Homoeopathic Medical College of Pennsylvania, which was to remain the center of homeopathic education in the United States.

Hering is known as the father of American homeopathy, not only because he set up the first homeopathic school in the United States, but also because of his valuable scientific researches and writings. The story of Hering's conversion to homeopathy goes back to his younger years in Germany. A publisher had approached Hering's medical mentor, a fervent antihomeopath named Robbi, to write a book demolish-

1. Much of the material in this section is derived from Harris Coulter, *Divided Legacy: A History of the Schism in Medical Thought*, 3 vols. (Washington, D.C.: McGrath Publishing Co., 1973), vol. 3.

ing the homeopathic doctrine. Because the elder physician was too busy to accept the assignment, he turned it over to the young Hering. Hering undertook a careful study of Hahnemann's writings, testing the instructions for drug provings, and the results convinced him of the validity of Hahnemann's doctrine. The publisher, Baumgartner, was so impressed by Hering's enthusiasm that he ended up publishing materials in favor of the New School, including a homeopathic journal.

Before moving to the United States, Hering spent eleven years doing scientific research with a Saxon government legation in Surinam, or Dutch Guiana, in South America, where he conducted the famous proving of *Lachesis* mentioned in chapter 6 and where he successfully applied homeopathic principles in the practice of medicine.

Hering was also the author of the *Domestic Physician,* the first homeopathic materia medica published in this country. The work was sold with a set of about forty homeopathic remedies, at first identified only by number to prevent their misuse, with instructions as to what number remedy to use for what symptom complex. This "homeopathic kit" contributed greatly to the spread of homeopathy by placing the medicines and the directions for their use directly in the hands of families who could thus treat their ailments in the absence of a homeopathic physician.

Other Nonorthodox Schools and the Lay Movement

Indeed, it was the lay movement in medicine that was a significant factor in the spread of homeopathy—as well as other dissenting systems—in the early decades of the nineteenth century. Increasingly disillusioned with the heroic practices and toxic drugs of orthodox medicine, the American public was a fertile field for the growth of new doctrines. A loosely knit school of "herb doctors," taking their cue from the American Indians' use of native plants, spread the use of herbal remedies. Most of these herbalists were laymen with no medical training; some were physicians who were known as botanical practitioners. Another dissenting sect was founded by Samuel Thomson, a New Hampshire farmer who schooled himself in herbal lore. Thomson's treatment initially consisted of steam baths and large doses of the herb Lobelia, and eventually the Thomsonians used over sixty-five herbal remedies. The Thomsonian system was patented, and the rights to practice it were sold; the system had its own infirmaries, pharmacies, and wholesale drug outlets. In 1838 Thomson claimed three million followers, or one-sixth of the nation's population, and in 1845 the herbalists and Thomsonians, united by their common reliance on medicinal herbs, organized the Eclectic Medical Institute, with other eclectic medical colleges being established in the years that followed.

With the spread of such medical doctrines, the regular physicians began to feel some alarm. Homeopathy, initially dismissed as a small heretical cult that would soon die a natural death, began to make great inroads on the clientele of regular medicine. Homeopaths appealed directly to the public to abandon allopathy and turn to the new doctrine for treatment of their ills; and lay practitioners, most of them women, who were aided by their books and kits of remedies, contributed to the spread of the New School through their ministrations to the sick in their communities.

But homeopathy was attracting not only the urban poor and those far from professional medical help in rural areas. Possibly because of its spiritual, vitalistic orientation, clergymen were attracted to the new doctrine and helped to proselytize it among their congregations. The wealthy and educated classes in the cities followed suit, and soon the allopaths began to fear that the entire intellectual, social, and business elite of the nation were converting to homeopathy.

Furthermore, homeopaths were generally earning far more attractive incomes than their allopathic counterparts. With the relatively limited supply of homeopathic practitioners and the privileged status of many of their patients, homeopaths could command higher fees and enjoy busier practices, and the allopaths began to recognize that homeopathy posed a serious threat.

As the numbers of homeopathic physicians increased, it became imperative that a national organization be formed—to uphold the high standards of practice of the New School and to continue scientific investigation into the materia medica. The American Institute of Homeopathy was founded in Philadelphia in 1844—the first national medical organization in the United States. The new institute attempted to insure high standards among practicing homeopaths by restricting admission to those who had received a complete allopathic medical education.

With the establishment of the institute, the field of homeopathy became the spearhead of the growing opposition to allopathy in the United States.

Allopathic Criticism of Homeopathy: An Examination of Holmes's Attack

As the allopaths lost their patients and their incomes to the homeopaths and other nonorthodox practitioners, they mounted a serious counterattack. They accounted for the desertion of their patients by pointing to the ignorance of the public, and attempted to discredit their dissenting competitors by charging them with inadequate education and quackery.

During the years just preceding and following the founding of the American Institute of Homeopathy, there was a flood of allopathic literature attacking the New School. The best known of these attacks is an essay by the famed physician-author-Supreme Court Justice Oliver Wendell Holmes, entitled "Homeopathy and Its Kindred Delusions," which was originally delivered before the Boston Society for the Diffusion of Useful Knowledge in 1842.[2] Although not scientifically and philosophically oriented, he was a witty master essayist, and humor effectively employed can be a very powerful weapon.

Although the underlying concepts of homeopathy may strike us as reasonable and of great significance, we must remember that our scientific knowledge has not yet progressed to the point that such notions as the ultramolecular

2. This essay appears in several collections of Holmes's writings. Page numbers cited herein are from "Homeopathy and Its Kindred Delusions," in *Medical Essays, 1842–1882* (Boston and New York: Houghton, Mifflin, 1895), pp 1–102.

dose are immediately plausible or disprovable. Holmes might equally have made fun of the idea that a mere handful of a radioactive substance could demolish an entire city, or that pictures could be transmitted through the air to our living room. Until our understanding of the inner workings of the human organism is more complete, it is healthy to be able to leaven our ignorance with humor.

The Founding of the American Medical Association and the Ban on Consultation

Reacting to the spread of homeopathy and other dissenting medical doctrines, the allopaths began to mount a full-scale attack. The allopaths had already lost their privileged position in the medical community as state legislatures had one by one eliminated licensing requirements restricting the practice of medicine to graduates of allopathic schools. Alternative medical schools were numerous by the 1840s, and in most states graduation from such institutions constituted a license to practice. One of the purported motives for the creation of a national allopathic organization was the need for "reform" in medical education—a code phrase meaning that dissenting schools should not be allowed to turn out licensed practitioners. Admittedly, some of the schools had low standards, but this applied as much to the substandard allopathic schools as to inferior alternative schools. Because the allopathic colleges exerted considerable influence on the policies of allopathic organizations, no serious effort at reform of the schools was undertaken throughout the nineteenth century.

In 1846, at the first National Medical Convention, the American Medical Association (AMA) was created. In addition to paying lip service to the need for improvement in education in the allopathic medical schools, the AMA launched a publicity campaign aimed at turning the public away from alternative forms of medicine. The 1847 Medical Convention adopted a Code of Ethics that prohibited its members from consulting with homeopaths.

To secure its position as official arbiter of medical opinion, the AMA required that local and state medical societies purge themselves of homeopathic members as a condition of their representation in the national organization. There ensued a period of witch-hunting among the allopathic profession as suspected sympathizers with the homeopathic doctrine were weeded out; even purchasing milk sugar at a homeopathic pharmacy was considered grounds for expulsion of a member from the AMA. For all practical purposes, communication between allopaths and homeopaths ceased, at least on an overt level, for the remainder of the nineteenth century. The AMA's Code of Ethics had the apparently unethical effect of jeopardizing the health of the patient, for a homeopath was not allowed to consult with an allopathic surgeon, for example, if his patient appeared to be in desperate need of surgical intervention; nor could the allopath receive referrals from his homeopathic colleagues, an economic situation that eventually led to clandestine contacts between the two schools.

Homeopathic Influences in the Nineteenth Century

Despite the AMA's efforts to bar communication between its members and the New School, the example of homeopathy had considerable influence over allopathic practice during the latter half of the nineteenth century. Regular medical doctors began to abandon the practice of bloodletting, partially owing to the homeopathic example in the use of aconite. The notion of the healing power of nature was revived in some allopathic circles. A few efforts were made to determine the action of allopathic drugs through provings on healthy subjects, but without a principle for the application of such findings, the knowledge was not widely used. Many drugs introduced or revived by the homeopaths were taken over into the allopathic pharmacopoeia.

Meanwhile, during the two decades following the Civil War, homeopathy enjoyed its greatest influence. Homeopathic sympathizers occupied important positions in government, and homeopaths gained wide acceptance in the public health service, the military, and other public institutions. In contrast with the AMA's policy of excluding women and blacks from the practice of medicine, the homeopaths became identified with the causes of Negro and female emancipation. There was an extensive network of homeopathic hospitals and institutions for the mentally ill, and even insurance companies recognized the benefits of homeopathic treatment. Gradually the homeopaths began to gain a sort of unofficial recognition among significant portions of the allopathic community; homeopathy became a lucrative form of practice, and with wide public and limited professional acceptance, the homeopaths for the first time enjoyed relatively easy and comfortable practices.

Division among the Homeopaths

During the years of its greatest prestige in the United States, homeopathy was increasingly troubled by division among its ranks. There had always been disagreement about the strictness with which Hahnemann's principles should be applied, and by 1880 the dispute became so marked that a new organization, the International Hahnemannian Association, was formed, its members withdrawing from the American Institute of Homeopathy and establishing a separate organization to uphold the purist point of view.

According to strict Hahnemannian principles, the practice of homeopathy is a difficult and time-consuming task. The temptation to take shortcuts had been present since the early days of the New School in Germany. Moreover, from the outset, many allopathic physicians—who had converted to homeopathy because of its success in epidemics—were never able to abandon competely their prior medical orientation.

One of the principal points of dispute was the question of the high potencies. The purists in homeopathy came to be kown as the high-potency practitioners, and the revisionists as low-potency physicians. Of course the division revolved around other issues as well. The "lows," as well as limiting their prescribing to the low-potency range, tended to move away from prescribing strictly on the basis of rigid similarity. They began to bring back the concept of the disease entity and to prescribe routinely on the basis of pathological diagnosis rather than on an exhaustive study of the patient's symptoms. This trend was reinforced by the coming into vogue of the germ theory of disease, which gave the "lows" further reason for abandoning the essential precepts of homeopathy. Because they were prescribing on the basis of pathological diagnosis, the "lows" began to prescribe larger doses, and they also began to combine medicines, rather than following the principle of the single remedy. Rather than drawing on the entire materia medica, many homeopaths tended to limit the number of remedies they employed to a relatively few familiar mainstays.

Such departures from strict Hahnemannian principles are not difficult to understand. As homeopaths found it necessary to see increasing numbers of patients—particularly as they moved from rural practices as "family doctors" to urban practices with transient patient populations—the temptation to take shortcuts in case taking and prescribing was strong. Many of the low-potency practitioners became specialists—reflecting the same trend in allopathic practice—and thus moved away from the cardinal principle of treating the patient as a whole.

The degree to which revisionism had weakened the homeopathic movement is reflected in the fact that when the high-potency physicians founded the International Hahnemannian Association in 1880, they could attract only seventy or eighty members out of the estimated ten thousand physicians who called themselves homeopaths.[3]

The Defeat of Homeopathy

The bickering within the ranks of homeopathy had seriously weakened the New School toward the end of the nineteenth century. Since so many homeopaths had strayed from the essential elements of Hahnemann's doctrine, the public was having a hard time distinguishing between homeopathy and allopathy. It only remained for modern economic and political forces to complete allopathy's triumph.

The modern pharmaceutical industry must receive a substantial share of the credit. Toward the end of the nine-

3. Coulter, *Divided Legacy*, 3:334.

teenth century, the newly flourishing drug companies gained the blessings of the allopathic profession, flooding the market with vast quantities of "proprietary" medications, whose names and/or composition were protected by law. Such remedies made the average physician's task much easier: no longer having to bother with pharmacology or exhaustive studies of their cases, doctors merely prescribed on the basis of the indications provided by the manufacturers of the drugs. The pharmaceutical industry poured huge sums of money into the AMA in the form of advertising in its journal and supported numerous other allopathic publications.

The AMA, strengthened by its alliance with the drug industry, began its final move to co-opt homeopathy by permitting state and local medical societies to abandon the old code of ethics and admit homeopaths as members. There followed a drive to recruit homeopaths and eclectics to allopathic organizations. Finally, in 1903, the AMA revised its national Code of Ethics, dropping the infamous consultation ban, but adding a new section:

It is inconsistent with the principles of medical science, and it is incompatible with honorable standing in the profession for physicians to designate their practice as based on an exclusive dogma or a sectarian system of medicine.[4]

Attracted by the apparent promise of a new respectability, many homeopaths joined the AMA and its subsidiary organizations, only to discover that they were not to be provided a forum for the discussion of their views. While homeopaths as individuals continued to enjoy lucrative practices, the homeopathic organizations became weaker as their members joined the allopathic camp.

Meanwhile, the homeopathic medical colleges were in trouble; they were not able to fill all the available openings or to turn out enough graduates to meet the increasing demand for homeopathic physicians. And many of the schools, since they were under the control of the "low-potency" faction, were not teaching Hahnemannian homeopathy.

4. *Journal of the American Medical Association* 40 (1903): 1379; quoted in Coulter, *Divided Legacy*, 3:434.

The homeopathic educational system was delivered the final blow when the AMA began in earnest its campaign for the reform of medical education. With overcrowding in the allopathic profession, there was an economic motive to reduce the number of licensed physicians. The institution of state licensing examinations in the 1880s and 1890s had demonstrated that many medical schools of all persuasions were turning out graduates who were poorly qualified in the basic sciences, and in 1904 the AMA's Committee on Medical Education established a set of standards for rating medical schools—standards that emphasized the allopathic orientation in the prescribed curriculum and facilities. AMA representatives visited all medical schools in 1907—including the homeopathic and eclectic colleges—and many schools complained about the poor ratings they received. The Council (Committee) on Medical Education therefore turned to an "objective" outside authority, the Carnegie Endowment for the Advancement of Teaching, to help with the project. In 1910 Abraham Flexner, representing the Carnegie Endowment, issued a report on his survey of the nation's medical schools. Guided by the criteria provided by the AMA (based on the curriculum of Johns Hopkins Medical School), the Flexner Report reflected a distinct bias against homeopathic colleges, as well as giving deservedly poor ratings to admittedly poor schools of all orientations. The effects were far-reaching. State examining boards began to bar the graduates of low-rated schools from taking licensing exams; the extensive private funding of medical schools was diverted to those schools receiving high ratings.

The homeopathic schools began to close or to convert to allopathic teaching. Of the twenty-two homeopathic colleges in 1900, only seven remained by 1918. In the ensuing years, these all ceased homeopathic instruction, the last to go being the Hahnemann Medical College of Philadelphia, in the 1930s. The International Hahnemannian Association, the upholders of pure Hahnemannian practice, went out of existence in 1957, and its remaining members merged with the American Institute of Homeopathy.

During this period, allopathic medicine had taken giant

strides. Many of the more dangerous practices of earlier times had been abandoned, and certain areas of allopathy, such as surgery, had achieved a high level of sophistication. The introduction of "miracle drugs" had made the treatment of many troublesome diseases easier and more certain—a mixed blessing, for it meant that the physician had to pay less attention to each patient. In addition, the drugs themselves were to prove to have unexpected side effects.

Although modern medicine had apparently made great advances in the direction of being more scientific, the shape of modern medical practice was determined to a large extent by economic and political factors that had little to do with concern for the patient and the treatment of illness. It was in the interests of the drug industry to sell as many of its products as possible, and spurred by widespread advertising campaigns and other inducements, both the general public and the medical profession made more and more liberal use of the new drugs.

Harris Coulter describes this situation as peculiar to the United States:

Adoption of the recommendations of the Flexner Report, the consequent restructuring of medical education along German laboratory lines, the alliance between the medical profession and the luxuriant American drug industry, and the increasing affluence of the American physician have combined to place a stamp on medicine in this country which distinguishes it from every other country in the world. It has become highly technical, highly business-dominated, highly politicized, and highly unpopular with the patient.[5]

The American public, as consumers of medical care, are not entirely without blame. Our nation's obsession with newer, more complex, and more expensive things has certainly been a contributing factor to the direction that medicine has taken. With the growth of tax-supported health care and prepaid insurance, every American feels entitled to the most highly sophisticated, expensive treatment available. It is not always the doctor who pushes unnecessary surgery and excessive drugging—the American patient demands these as his right. As we have observed, it is only with the developing aware-

5. Coulter, *Divided Legacy*, 3:499.

ness of the dangers of highly technologized society that the American public is becoming aware of the related dangers of assembly-line technological medicine.

HOMEOPATHY TODAY IN THE UNITED STATES

The present status of homeopathy in the United States is defined by four factors: (1) the existence of a relatively small number of licensed homeopathic physicians whose practices reflect a wide range of attitudes toward the application of homeopathic principles; (2) the absence of formal homeo- pathic medical education in this country since the 1930s; (3) the growing interest among the lay public in alternative medicine, specifically in homeopathy; and (4) the attempt by young, recently graduated physicians to obtain training in the principles and practice of homeopathy.

The Professional Homeopathic Community

The American Institute of Homeopathy, founded in 1844, was the first national medical organization in the United States. Its membership comprises licensed medical profes- sionals (M.D.'s, osteopaths, and dentists) who employ the methodology of homeopathy in their practices. The *Journal of the American Institute of Homeopathy* is the organiza- tion's official publication, and it appears quarterly.

The National Center for Homeopathy, in Washington, D.C., is an organization composed of physicians and non- physicians whose Board of Directors reflects that tradition. It was incorporated to preserve and promote homeopathy through the appropriate education and training of the lay and the professional public, the sale and publication of ho- meopathic literature, the sponsorship of homeopathic research, and the fulfillment of other services. The National Center also serves as the business office for the American Institute of Homeopathy and for the American Board of Homeo- therapeutics.

Since its separate incorporation from the American Foun- dation for Homeopathy in 1974, predicated on an IRS ruling, the National Center for Homoepathy has provided most of the public information and promotional activities in the U.S. It has published a *Directory of Homeopathic Practitioners*, sponsored many public seminars, convened an instructive Annual Conference, offered an annual professional training course and published an informative monthly newsletter.

A new organization, the International Foundation for the Promotion of Homeopathy (IFPH), has recently been providing most of the public promotional services in the form of referral service for classical homeopaths, public lectures and seminars, professional conferences, training courses for professionals, and an informative newsletter.

We have noted that the professional homeopathic community in this country has dwindled from approximately one-sixth of the medical profession in 1900 to a few hundred at present. Although interest in homeopathy has been increasing during the past decade, membership in the professional organizations remains small. An obvious contributing factor in the lag between public demand and the supply of homeopathic physicians is that there is at present not a single homeopathic medical school in this country. A substantial proportion of the membership in the AIH and the state organizations consists of homeopaths who received their medical education in the 1930s and earlier; younger members have either been educated abroad or have obtained their training in this country through other channels.

Since many homeopathic physicians received their education abroad, they may follow slightly different practices than their American-trained colleagues. For example, in France it is common practice for the homeopath to prescribe at the same time a chronic remedy in high potency and one or more "drainage" remedies in low potency, an obvious deviation from the Hahnemannian principles of the single remedy.

Thus the licensed physicians in this country are practicing homeopathy in a variety of ways, reflecting differences in generations, the places where they received their training, and their personal convictions about the proper application of the homeopathic doctrine. In an interview in 1978, Dr. Frederic Schmid, then president of the American Institute of Homeopathy, stresses that such differences in therapeutic approach should not take precedence over a common dedication to the basic principles of the homeopathic doctrine, for it is only through unity that homeopathy can survive.

The Homeopathic Lay Movement

The major impetus for the spread of awareness about homeopathy as an alternative to orthodox medicine has come from the rapidly expanding homeopathic lay movement. The American Institute of Homeopathy embraces a wide range of approaches to the application of the homeopathic doctrine, but the lay movement is generally concerned with the promotion of pure Hahnemannian homeopathy. Across the United States, lay study groups, or groups comprising both laypeople and licensed professionals, are going deeply into the homeopathic philosophy and materia medica and learning the principles of homeopathic prescribing in its classical form— the single remedy, careful case taking, strict repertorization, the uses of high potencies, and the like. The existence of serious organized groups of laypeople studying homeopathy has two important results: (1) it is largely through the efforts of such laypeople that the homeopathic analysis of health and disease and the Hahnemannian principles of treatment are being promulgated among the general public; and (2) the purist orientation of the lay groups holds up a mirror in which the practice of homeopathy by licensed professionals can be measured. Thus the lay groups serve a valuable educational function for the consumers of health care.

It is only natural that members of lay study groups would want to begin to apply the homeopathic principles that they have learned in treating illness. The official position of the National Center for Homeopathy is that laypeople should limit themselves to the study of homeopathic principles and philosophy and to the use of homeopathy in first aid, and that all other problems should remain within the domain of the homeopathic physician. In reality, however, there are a number of lay homeopaths practicing in this country. The Hering Family Health Clinic in Berkeley, California, has a staff composed of both M.D.'s and lay prescribers; in such a setting, the lay homeopaths have the legal and ethical safeguard of working in a paraprofessional capacity under the auspices of licensed professionals who are available for consultation. Other lay prescribers may work in a licensed physician's office, seeing their own clientele, or they may have independent practices. Because of the legal restrictions in most states, independent lay homeopaths must be careful to define the limits of the services they offer, and of course must refer their clients to licensed physicians whenever indicated. The entire question of lay prescribing is rather ambiguous at the present time. The National Center for Homeopathy does not officially recognize the practice of homeopathy by lay prescribers who may have been applying Hahnemann's principles in a clinical setting for many years. Of course there is justification for the concern that incompetent lay prescribers give all of homeopathy a bad name. Given the realities of the situation, it might be useful for the organized homeopathic community to put some thought into an effort at self-regulation, whereby standards of practice would be established and lay prescribers examined for their competence to consult with patients within clearly defined limits.

Homeopathic Education

The aspiring homeopath in this country must attend a regular four-year medical school and put in a year of internship in order to qualify for licensing in the state in which he wants to practice. By that time, having had extensive exposure to allopathic assumptions and attitudes, the young physician may find it difficult to readjust his thinking to the homeopathic approach. Once the conventional allopathic qualifications are met, a physician can go on to obtain training in homeopathy as a specialty. But such training is relatively unavailable in the United States. "Every summer since 1924, the National Center for Homeopathy has been sponsoring a summer school in Millersville, Pennsylvania. There is a course which introduces licensed professionals to the history, principles, and materia medica of homeopathy; there are also courses for dentists, veterinarians, and nurses. A separate course is offered for laypeople, with the emphasis on philosophy rather than practice, except for homeopathic first aid.

Obviously, a three-week curriculum is not sufficient. The mastery of the materia medica alone can occupy years of regular lectures and private study. Furthermore, it is only through clinical experience under the guidance of a competent homeopath that the newcomer can really begin to grasp the subtleties of correct prescribing. Thus, physicians who receive their first homeopathic training at Millersville must undertake to further their education through other means.

Some physicians go abroad to study at the homeopathic schools in London, Vienna, and other European cities; or they go to Mexico or India. In Athens, Greece, George Vithoulkas has gathered an international group of physicians who are obtaining clinical training under his guidance. This training is now being done under the auspices of the International Foundation for the Promotion of Homeopathy, recently founded by George Vitholkas and by Dr. Bill Gray of California. Besides its work in Greece, the foundation offered its first one-year homeopathic training program in California in 1980. A group of 18 licensed physicians completed the course, which consisted of instruction by Dr. Gray for most of the year, with advanced seminars conducted by Vithoulkas at the end of the year.

The Foundation hopes that physicians who complete the one-year training program will eventually be able to become faculty members at a five-year medical college in California which will provide a complete education in homeopathic medicine parallel to the instruction in a regular medical school. Backers of this plan are optimistic that such a medical college can be set up in California, and that its graduates will be eligible for licensing by the state. The address of IFPH headquarters is 4 Sherman Avenue, Fairfax, CA 94930 (phone 415-457-8758).

Aside from such formal educational opportunities, the young American physician may be able to join the practice of an experienced homeopath who serves as preceptor. Once the young allopath has learned the rudiments of homeopathic theory, such an arrangement can help him to progress rapidly in his mastery of homeopathy in clinical practice, as well as relieving the work load of the busy seasoned prescriber.

Regardless of how homeopathic education might develop, the essential ingredient for the training of competent homeopathic physicians is the availability of experienced masters to set an example in practice and to communicate to their students their deep understanding of the homeopathic doctrine and the materia medica. Each summer, the IFPH offers a two-week introductory course held at University of California Campus at Berkeley, California. Taught by IFPH-trained classical homeopaths, this course balances classical theory with practical teaching of first aid and acute prescribing. The IFPH also conducts an intensive, one-year training course for licensed health professionals. Offered on alternate years on either the West or East Coast, this course consists of five one-week sessions spaced two months apart, culminated by a two- or four-week advanced session with George Vithoulkas. This course is the most advanced offered currently in the United States.

OTHER COUNTRIES

Homeopathy is more widespread in other countries than it is in the United States. Americans traveling abroad note that in many European cities the homeopathic pharmacy is as commonplace as our corner drugstore.

England is an important center of homeopathic teaching and practice, and homeopathic physicians and hospitals are part of the National Health Service. Other Commonwealth nations, notably Australia, New Zealand, and Canada, also have many practicing homeopaths.

Hahnemann spent his last years in Paris, and France continues to be a stronghold of homeopathy. The doctrine remains strong in Germany; Switzerland and Holland have significant numbers of practitioners; and Vienna has a highly regarded teaching program. Reportedly homeopathy is also widely practiced in the Soviet Union.

India has the largest number of homeopaths of any country in the world; according to a 1972 government estimate there were 300,000 full-time homeopaths in India, of whom 70,000 were registered by state boards, and the balance were ineligible for state qualification. Homeopathy is officially recognized and supported by the Indian government as a separate system of medicine. In recent years the nation's homeopathic teaching institutions have been recognized to ensure that students receive a thorough medical education. At present there are some forty homeopathic medical colleges in India, offering four- or six-year programs. India is also the most active nation in the publishing of homeopathic literature, much of it consisting of reprints in English of basic homeopathic texts.

The Latin-American countries also have substantial numbers of homeopathic practitioners; Mexico has several schools, and homeopathic doctors can be found throughout the country.

In 1925, the International Homeopathic League held its first meeting in Holland, and the organization has remained active ever since. Among its aims are the establishment of uniform standards for the preparation and potentization of homeopathic remedies, the reporting of research, and the maintenance of an international community of homeopaths— of great importance for those who practice in relative isolation in countries where homeopathy is a minority doctrine.

Despite the setbacks suffered in this country, homeopathy appears to be entering a new period of growth. But can a system formulated some 170 years ago stand up to modern allopathic medicine in terms of scientific soundness? Let us turn to an examination of homeopathy in terms of its scientific procedures and the verifiability of its doctrine under laboratory conditions.

9

THE FUTURE OF HOMEOPATHY

In order to evaluate the impact that homeopathy may have in the years to come, we must examine a number of factors that affect both the demand for homeopathic treatment and the supply.

THE DEMAND FOR ALTERNATIVE HEALTH CARE

The time seems to be ripe for a large-scale revival of interest in homeopathy. The rising costs of orthodox health care, the increase in iatrogenic illness, the new epidemics of chronic diseases and mental illness, as well as the leisure to think about every ache and pain are all causing large numbers of people to reexamine their attitudes toward medical care and to search for approaches that are gentler and more in tune with the natural healing processes of the human organism. With the spread of the "growth movement" in the United States, people are consciously cultivating their own abilities to take initiative in the regulation of their mental and physical well-being. The concerns expressed by environmentalists about the indiscriminate application of modern technology are mirrored in the health field, and there has been an attempt to find ways of treating illness that are less disruptive of the human organism and its relationship with the external world. Thus economic, philosophical, and scientific motives are combining to promote a holistic view of man in his environment and of the human organism as a vital self-healing being.

THE HOMEOPATHIC COMMUNITY

As people explore alternatives to orthodox medical care, it is likely that there will be an increased demand for homeopathic treatment. The supply of competent homeopathic practitioners in this country is limited. Some young physicians, disillusioned with allopathic medicine, will respond to the demand for homeopathy by studying its principles and beginning to apply it in their practices, but there is also a real danger that many unqualified homeopathic practitioners will attempt to fill the gap by offering their services to the public. Homeopaths fear that the practice of homeopathy by people who are not sufficiently versed in its principles—or not sufficiently dedicated to apply these principles in the strictest, most conscientious manner—will endanger patients as well as discrediting homeopathy as a whole.

For this reason it must be a first priority in the homeopathic community to make sure that anyone who wants to become a homeopathic practitioner will be able to receive adequate training and will be able to obtain clinical experience by working alongside thoroughly competent and committed master prescribers. How such education will be provided is not clear at this time. Some aspiring homeopaths may go abroad to study under the masters in other countries. Others will attend short courses here in the United States and then join the practices of experienced homeopaths who will show them how homeopathy is properly practiced in a clinical setting.

The homeopathic physicians in this country have a tremendous responsibility to set an example, both for younger doctors who are beginning to apply homeopathy in their practices and for the public at large, who will only know what homeopathy can accomplish if they can see the results of proper prescribing. Homeopaths at present are somewhat reluctant to publicize the potential power of their system, for they realize that in most parts of this country people are not able to obtain competent homeopathic treatment, even if they are convinced that it is the best approach. But if the homeopathic analysis of the causes of chronic diseases and the dangers of allopathic treatment is correct, then it is the responsibility of homeopaths to inform the public of the existence of an option and to disseminate enough information so that the intelligent consumer of health care will be able to differentiate between correct prescribing and incompetent application of the homeopathic doctrine.

THE PHILOSOPHICAL ORIENTATION OF HOMEOPATHY

Although homeopathy is theoretically able to cure any disease in which there is not serious organic damage, it incorporates an attitude toward health that will not be immediately acceptable to some people.

In our modern world, it has sometimes seemed that total freedom from discomfort, that age-old goal of humanity, was almost within our grasp. Many of the new allopathic drugs have produced spectacular results in the relief of pain, anxiety, and functional disorders, and many people have become dependent on such suppressive and palliative medicines, preferring to obtain immediate relief no matter what the cost in the long run. Some allopathic medicines deaden the sensations of the patient; the symptoms may still be there, but the patient does not feel them. Skin eruptions and other "cosmetically unacceptable" symptoms can often be suppressed through allopathic treatment, although the conditions that gave rise to such problems may continue unabated. Given the attitudes instilled in our culture through the mass media and the popular glorification of youth and beauty, it is understandable that people would be reluctant to undertake a form of treatment that promised no immediate resolution of the external and superficial manifestations of disease, regardless of how beneficial that therapeutic approach might be on the innermost levels of the human organism.

We have seen that, in theory and in practice, homeopathy may involve temporary discomfort for the patient. As successive layers of the patient's miasmatic pattern are peeled away, symptoms will reappear, and they may be exceedingly troublesome. Homeopaths point out that, if a remedy is properly selected, throughout these sufferings the patient will feel better in himself. Homeopathy places higher value on the innermost parts of man than on the transitory expressions of disturbances on the surface, but there are some people who would "rather die" than experience an unattractive skin eruption in the course of treatment. Such patients cannot be expected to cooperate with homeopathic treatment; unless they can undergo a radical change in their attitudes, they are likely to suppress surface symptoms that must come out while cure is in progress.

From earliest time, humanity has had to confront suffering on both a practical and a philosophical level. Ritualistic suffering, in the form of sacrifice and personal self-denial, has from the dawn of humanity been a mechanism in the appeasement of inferred hostile external forces and in the movement toward the perfectibility of the human organism and of society. Freud's formulation of the theory of psychoanalysis holds that as the patient explores the repressed material in his psyche, unpleasant and traumatic events from the past come to the surface, and by reexperiencing the suffering associated with the traumas, the patient clears himself emotionally. Among the contemporary holistic therapies, such techniques as Rolfing involve considerable discomfort for the patient, but, experiencing such discomfort, the patient is able to unlearn the destructive postural and muscular habits that have distorted his bodily functions.

It would appear that at this stage of our evolution we cannot hope to be free of pain and suffering. Perhaps the attempt to mask this pain, to narcotize ourselves physically and mentally, is actually doing us further damage. Perhaps we ought to remember that pain and suffering are part of life for most people on our planet. Material wealth may *not* offer the joyride so many of us seem to demand, nor will it give us a life that transcends the zoological order.

Although such homeopaths as Kent have gone so far as to say that man's susceptibility to disease is a reflection of his imperfection on the spiritual plane, homeopathy is by and large an extremely optimistic medical science, believing that the organism *is* perfectible—that through proper medical treatment, combined with correct living, it is possible for us to reach a state of health, happiness, and freedom. The road to such health may not be completely smooth: homeopathic treatment may involve the patient in real physical discomfort in the course of cure. It is almost as if the patient must expiate his and his forefathers' "sin" of "getting off easy" in the suppressive treatment of previous illnesses.

The former patient of a noted homeopathic physician in New York recounted a story that illustrates the philosophical orientation of Hahnemann's doctrine. Her entire family was under the homeopath's care, and one of the children had recurrent bouts of tonsillitis. The mother and the homeopath both wanted to avoid tonsillectomy, but the little girl experienced a high fever and great discomfort with each attack. The mother kept calling the doctor, asking if she couldn't give her daughter aspirin to afford her some relief. The doctor told the mother, "There is no way you can save your daughter the experience of pain, nor would it be good for her." Twenty years later, the mother recalls the words of this doctor with great respect.

George Vithoulkas recently came from Greece to San Francisco to deliver a series of lectures to a group of some four hundred health professionals and laypeople. The event was noteworthy, not only because it demonstrated the growing interest in homeopathy among people who are exploring alternatives to traditional medicine, but also because it gave the audience a chance to experience the profound dedication of a master homeopath to the strict classical application of the homeopathic doctrine. Vithoulkas stressed that homeopathy, when properly practiced, can effect remarkable changes in the life and health of the patient. He summed up its potential by saying, "Homeopathy is such a deep and dynamic tool that it can really bring about a true revolution—the most peaceful revolution that the world has witnessed so far."

What are the dimensions of the revolution that Vithoulkas envisions? In his book, *Homoeopathy: Medicine of the New Man,* he quotes some remarks by Dr. W. H. Schwartz:

If someone had the genius to awaken the world and make it realize what homeopathy can do, it would mean a new epoch for humanity—a renaissance in medicine. Indeed, homeopathy is so far-reaching that its universal use in medicine would mean great progress toward the millennium, as homeopathy has to do with not only the physical but spiritual development in man—the homeopathic remedy actually saves souls in this way. It assists in destroying the evils by creating harmony of the physical organs and thus promoting a pure vehicle for intellect and spirit to function. Homeopathy helps to open the higher centres for spiritual and celestial influx. It is the only scientific system of medicine, but it is too difficult to master without intensive training.[1]

Is homeopathy a teleological system for the individual expiation of Original Sin? If such is the case, it is obviously not for everyone in this modern world, for many people will avoid suffering no matter what the ultimate cost. But for those who feel a deep and urgent need to know themselves, to confront their weaknesses and resolve them, homeopathy in conjunction with other practices may be a means of helping to remove the layers of ignorance, blindness, and selfishness that enshroud the individual psyche as it struggles to be free. In the final analysis, it seems as though a perfectly moral life may be the end aim of *all* therapies.

HOMEOPATHY AND THE REVOLUTION IN SCIENCE

We are all aware that the history of science over the last century reflects an almost exponential expansion of the frontiers of human knowledge. Revolutionary scientific discoveries, each with a potential significance equivalent to the discovery of the wheel, are coming upon us at an ever-accelerating pace. Witness such developments as Einstein's theories of relativity, the decoding of the DNA molecule, the growth of electronic communications, and the evolution of the science of cybernetics and the creation of the computer as a tool in the service of human intelligence. Despite the often mundane and sometimes outright destructive applica-

1. William Henry Schwartz, M.D., *Homoeopathy* 5 (1936): 15–18; quoted in George Vithoulkas, *Homoeopathy: Medicine of the New Man* (New York: Avon Books, 1971), p. 112.

tions of these scientific concepts, they all have something in common: they represent the expansion of human understanding into an area where purely materialistic reasoning is no longer relevant. Such concepts as electromagnetic radiation, matter-energy field theory, the binary logic of the computer, and the transmission of the genetic code through DNA show that our scientists have undergone a radical transformation in the way they understand the forces at work in our universe. Those who are working at the theoretical frontiers of their fields are becoming increasingly aware that there are things going on of which they are at present only dimly aware, and many are beginning to suspect that there may be more to some of the ancient wisdom of our race than meets the technological eye.

Although our technology sometimes seems to threaten to run wild and destroy the very human species that set it in motion, technology by definition remains human in its focus; it has been designed to serve man and to extend the limited potential of his physical body. At the frontiers of science, it becomes clear that there is a significant interface between the human organism and scientific theory—either because the nature of the human mind itself limits the kinds of knowledge that can be obtained or because ethical considerations arise when scientific discoveries (such as genetic engineering) reveal the potential for altering or even destroying the species that has acquired such knowledge.

Scientists in widely diverse disciplines therefore erect theoretical models of the human organism that will take such considerations into account. Where such models are lacking, questions must remain unanswered. Many of the unresolved issues in orthodox medicine reflect the absence of a unified theoretical model of the human organism. The pharmacologist theorizes about the action of psychoactive drugs at nerve receptor sites in terms of electrochemical reactions, but the theories break down when they fail to account for the way such reactions mediate the effects on human consciousness. Allopathic physicians treating terminal cases observe that there is some undefinable will to live that keeps some patients alive or even leads to their recovery; medicine has only the most rudimentary knowledge of what constitutes this will to live and how to reach it through pharmacology or psychotherapy.

Although homeopathy cannot presently explain such phenomena in terms that can be evaluated in laboratory experiments, it is noteworthy that the model of the human organism propounded by Hahnemann is not invalidated by the present state of scientific knowledge. Homeopathy defines wellness as the integrated, freely creative functioning of the mental, emotional, and physical spheres of the organism. The responses of these three spheres to the external environment are mediated by what Hahnemann called the vital force. Modern homeopaths conceive of this vital force in terms of an "electromagnetic" field—a field that can only be influenced by inputs as subtle as the field itself. Homeopaths speculate that potentized remedies acquire the same kinds of properties that are present in this field—that the energies inherent in medicinal substances are by some unknown process rendered sufficiently subtle to be able to establish a sort of "resonance" with the vital force, or field, of the susceptible individual. This most contemporary homeopathic model is consistent with the speculative models of the human organism that have been erected in other sciences, but it is even more significant that Hahnemann himself, without the benefit of the past 170 years of scientific progress, expressed the action of the remedies and the causes of disease in similar terms.

Our expanding scientific knowledge may eventually yield a revolution in human consciousness, in which humankind begins to understand the interaction of the human body, emotions, and mind in terms that are congruent with the homeopathic model. If such a revolution should occur, it is unlikely that even the mammoth pharmaceutical industry and organized orthodox medicine combined could hold back the tide of inquiry into a broader application of homeopathy and other alternative therapeutics in the treatment of human illness.

Homeopathy has always insisted that it is a purely empirical system of therapeutics. Despite various speculative models that have been erected to attempt to account for disease and the action of the remedies, no homeopath would pretend to know the nature of the energies at work. It is possible that homeopathy, as presently practiced, is only an approximation of what we will ultimately discover to be the best possible method for treating the sick and maintaining our health. Remedies may not need to be prepared by painstaking trituration and succussion; perhaps there is another way of imparting the energetic patterns to a neutral medium. Long and tedious case taking, based on the close observation of the physician and the verbal reports of the patient and his attendants, may someday be supplanted by direct measurement of the vital force—or electromagnetic field—through means we can only dimly conceive at present. Perhaps someday we will be able to cure our illnesses with almost perfect infallibility on an energetic level alone.

Such speculation can be confirmed or invalidated only with the passage of time. It is significant, however, that the homeopathic model has for some 170 years remained consistent with the ever-expanding body of scientific knowledge concerning the inner workings of the human organism. Current organized allopathic medicine dismisses homeopathy as an archaic doctrine. Thoughtful workers in the nonorthodox therapies repeatedly state that homeopathy is the medicine of the future. If homeopathy continues to attract dedicated, inquiring minds—practitioners as well as experimenters and theoreticians who keep abreast of developments in all areas of human knowledge—Hahnemann's doctrine may have a significant formative influence on the revolution in the health and sanity of our planet that mankind is yearning for.

APPENDIX A

FURTHER READINGS

BOOKS ON HOMEOPATHY

Many books on homeopathy are difficult to obtain. The ones listed below are available either through regular bookstores or through the sources listed in this appendix. The Indian editions of the basic homeopathic texts are most generally available; new Indian editions are being issued constantly, so many important homeopathic books may become more widely available in the future.

Titles followed with (I) are introductory in nature and do not presuppose any prior knowledge of homeopathy; they are generally addressed to the layperson. Books marked with two asterisks (**) are essential reading for serious students of homeopathy.

Allen, H. C., M.D. *Keynotes and Characteristics with Comparisons of Some of the Leading Remedies of the Materia Medica.* 6th Indian ed. New Delhi: Jain Publishing Co., 1977.

Blackie, Margery G. *The Patient, Not the Cure.* London: Macdonald and Jane's, 1976. (I)

**Boericke, William, M.D. *Pocket Manual of Homeopathic Materia Medica.* 9th ed. New York: Boericke and Runyon, Inc., 1927.

**Coulter, Harris L. *Homoeopathic Medicine.* Washington, D.C.: American Foundation of Homoeopathy, 1972.

————. *Divided Legacy: A History of the Schism in Medical Thought. Volume I: The Patterns Emerge: Hippocrates to Paracelsus. Volume II: Progress and Regress: J. B. Van Helmont to Claude Bernard. Volume III: Science and Ethics in American Medicine, 1800–1914.* Washington, D.C.: Wehawken Book Co., 1973.

————. *Homeopathic Influences in Nineteenth-Century Allopathic Therapeutics.* Washington, D.C.: American Institute of Homeopathy, 1973.

Gallavardin, Dr. *How to Cure Alcoholism.* Translated by Irenaeus D. Foulon, and foreword by Jack Cooper, M.D. Katonah, N.Y.: East-West Arts, Ltd., 1976.

**Gibson, D. M. *First Aid Homeopathy in Accidents and Ailments.* 6th ed. London: British Homoeopathic Association, 1977.

Haehl, Richard. *Samuel Hahnemann: His Life and Work.* 2 vols. London: Homoeopathic Publishing Co., 1922.

**Hahnemann, Samuel. *The Chronic Diseases (Theoretical Part).* Translated from the second enlarged German edition of 1835 by Prof. Louis H. Tafel. New Delhi: Jain Publishing Co., 1976.

**————. *Organon of Medicine.* Translated with preface by William Boericke, M.D., and introduction by James Krauss, M.D. Indian edition. New Delhi: B. Jain Publishers, 1976.

**Hubbard-Wright, Elizabeth, M.D. *A Brief Study Course in Homoeopathy.* St. Louis, Mo.: Formur, Inc., 1977.

**Kent, James Tyler, A.M., M.D. *Lectures on Homoeopathic Materia Medica.* 1st Indian ed. New Delhi: Jain Publishing Co., 1972.

**————. *Lectures on Homoeopathic Philosophy.* New Delhi: B. Jain Publishers, 1974.

**_____. *New Remedies, Clinical Cases, Lesser Writings, Aphorisms and Precepts.* New Delhi: B. Jain Publishers, 1976.

**_____. *Repertory of the Homoeopathic Materia Medica.* 3rd ed. Chicago: Ehrhart & Karl, 1924.

Panos, Maesimund B., M.D. *Homeopathic Medicine at Home.* Los Angeles: J. P. Tarcher, 1980.

**Roberts, Herbert A., M.D. *The Principles and Art of Cure by Homoeopathy.* New Delhi: B. Jain Publishers, 1976.

Shadman, A. *Who Is Your Doctor and Why?* Boston: House of Edinboro, 1958. (I)

**Sharma, C. H. *A Manual of Homoeopathy and Natural Medicine.* New York: E. P. Dutton & Co., Inc., 1975. (I)

**Shepherd, Dr. Dorothy. *Homoeopathy for the First Aider.* Devon, England: Health Science Press, 1977. (I)

_____. *Magic of the Minimum Dose.* Devon, England: Health Science Press, 1964. (I)

_____. *More Magic of the Minimum Dose.* Devon, England: Health Science Press, 1974. (I)

Sheppard, K. *The Treatment of Cats by Homoeopathy.* Devon, England: Health Science Press, 1960. (I)

_____. *The Treatment of Dogs by Homoeopathy.* Devon, England: Health Science Press, 1975. (I)

Stephenson, James H., M.D. *A Doctor's Guide to Helping Yourself with Homeopathic Remedies.* 1st British ed. Wellingborough, Northamptonshire, England: Thorsons Publishers Ltd., 1977. (I)

**Vithoulkas, George. *Homoeopathy: Medicine of the New Man*. New York: Avon Books, 1971. (I)

**_____. *The Science of Homeopathy*. New York: Grove Press, 1980.

**Wheeler, Charles S. *An Introduction to the Principles and Practice of Homoeopathy*. London: British Homoeopathic Association, 1920.

Whitmont, Edward C. *Psyche and Substance: Essays on Homeopathy in Light of Jungian Psychology*. Richmond, California: North Atlantic Books, 1980.

SOURCES OF HOMEOPATHIC BOOKS

For books that cannot be obtained through a local bookstore, the following suppliers carry relatively large stocks of books on homeopathy. Those marked with an asterisk will provide a book list on request, and they will handle mail orders; others may do so also if you inquire by mail.

Boericke & Tafel, Inc.*
1011 Arch Street
Philadelphia, PA 19107

John A. Borneman & Sons*
1208 Amosland Road
Norwood, PA 19074

East West Books
506 W. Diversey
Chicago, IL 60614

Ehrhart & Karl*
17 N. Wabash Avenue
Chicago, IL 60602

Formur, Inc.*
4200 Laclede Avenue
Saint Louis, MO 63108

Health Research
70 Lafayette Street
Mokelumne Hill, CA 95245

Hering Family Health Clinic
Suite 107, 2340 Ward Street
Berkeley, CA 94705

Homeopathic Educational
Services*
5916 Chabot Crest
Oakland, CA 94618
P.O. Box 5015
Berkeley, CA 94705
(Send self-addressed,
stamped envelope for
annotated book list.)

Humphreys Pharmacal Co.*
63 Meadow Road
Rutherford, NJ 07070

International Foundation for
the Promotion of
Homeopathy
4 Sherman Avenue
Fairfax, CA 94930

National Center for
Homoeopathy*
7810 Helena Drive
Falls Church, VA 22043

Sakti Distributors
320 State Street
Madison, WI 53703

Shambhala Books
2482 Telegraph Avenue
Berkeley, CA 94704

Standard Homoeopathic Co.*
436 W. Eighth Street
Los Angeles, CA 90014

Yes! Inc. Bookshop
1035 Thirty-first Street, N.W.
Washington, D.C. 20007

APPENDIX B

HOMEOPATHIC PHYSICIANS AND STUDY RESOURCES

HOMEOPATHIC PHYSICIANS

For a listing of homeopathic physicians arranged by state and city, write to the National Center for Homeopathy and request the *Directory of Homeopathic Practitioners*. The price of this publication is approximately $3.00. The address is:

National Center for Homeopathy
1500 Massachusetts Avenue, N.W.
Washington, D.C. 20005

The IFPH will also send a referral list of classical constitutional homeopaths for $1.00. IFPH address above.

HOMEOPATHIC STUDY GROUPS

For a listing of study groups, arranged by state, write to the National Center for Homeopathy and request their publication *Homoeopathic Study Groups*.

SUMMER PROGRAM

The National Center for Homoeopathy, at the above address, will provide on request a catalog of courses for its summer program at Millersville, Pennsylvania. Courses are offered for both licensed medical professionals and laypeople.

The National Center will also provide information concerning regional seminars throughout the year that are sponsored by the National Center for Instruction in Homeotherapeutics and that are open to physicians and medical students.

The IFPH offers a two-week introductory course for both professionals and qualified laypeople held at Stanford University.

TRAINING FOR HEALTH PROFESSIONALS

The International Foundation for Homeopathy offers training in homeopathy for licensed physicians.

National Center for Homeopathy offers training in homeopathy for licensed physicians, veterinarians, dentists, and nurses.

APPENDIX C

SUPPLIERS OF HOMEOPATHIC REMEDIES

The following pharmaceutical suppliers sell homeopathic remedies over the counter and by mail order. Firms marked with an asterisk are members of the American Association of Homeopathic Pharmacists, and they can supply mail-order catalogs on request. Many of these companies also sell homeopathic first aid kits. Homeopathic remedies are also becoming increasingly available at health food stores, and may be the most convenient source for commonly employed remedies in many communities.

Annandale Apothecary
7023 Little River Turnpike
Annandale, VA 22003

Boericke & Tafel, Inc.*
1011 Arch Street
Philadelphia, PA 19107

John A. Borneman & Sons*
1208 Amosland Road
Norwood, PA 19074

Ehrhart & Karl*
17 N. Wabash Avenue
Chicago, IL 60602

Horton & Converse
621 W. Pico Boulevard
Los Angeles, CA 90015

Humphreys Pharmacal Co.*
63 Meadow Road
Rutherford, NJ 07070

Kiehl Pharmacy, Inc.
109 Third Avenue
New York, NY 10003

Luyties Pharmacal
Company*
4200 Laclede Avenue
Saint Louis, MO 63108

Nutri-Dyn
110 Twentieth Street
Santa Monica, CA 90406

Santa Monica Drug
1513 Fourth Street
Santa Monica, CA 90401

Standard Homoeopathic
Pharmacy*
436 W. Eighth Street
Los Angeles, CA 90014

D. L. Thompson Homeopathic
Supplies
844 Yonge Street
Toronto 5, Ontario, CANADA

Washington Homeopathic
Pharmacy*
4914 Delray Avenue
Bethesda, MD 20014

Weleda, Inc.
841 S. Main Street,
P.O. Box 121
Spring Valley, NY 10977

GLOSSARY*

Acute disease. An illness or symptom having a relatively rapid onset and development and a relatively short course; opposite of CHRONIC DISEASE.

Aggravation. Increase in the intensity of a symptom or condition. May be the result of an environmental or psychic stimulus or of the administration of a drug. A homeopathic aggravation is an intensification of a patient's symptoms caused by the administration of a remedy that produces the same symptoms as are exhibited by the patient. Opposite of AMELIORATION.

Allopathy. Treatment of disease using drugs whose effects are different from those of the disease being treated; from the Greek *allos* ("different") and *pathein* ("disease, suffering"). The medicines employed bear no particular relationship to the symptoms being treated.

Amelioration. Decrease in the intensity of a symptom or condition as a result of external or psychic stimulus or the administration of a drug. Opposite of AGGRAVATION.

Antidote. To counteract or neutralize the action of a medicine.

Antimiasmatic. A remedy capable of producing the symptoms of a chronic MIASM; therefore, according to the Law of Similars, a remedy that can be used to remove the chronic miasm.

Antipsoric. A remedy capable of producing the symptoms of PSORA, and therefore used to treat the psoric miasm (see ANTIMIASMATIC).

* Words in small caps indicate cross reference.

Arndt-Schulz law. An observation in allopathic medicine that small drug doses kindle vital activities, moderate doses increase them, large doses depress them, and largest doses remove them.

Avogadro's number. The number of atoms in a gram atom or of molecules in a gram mole of any substance; a constant, equal to 6.023×10^{23}.

Case taking. Eliciting the patient's total symptoms, or variations from normal, through observation, examination, and recording of the patient's complaints, past history, family history, and physical examination.

Centesimal scale. A system of serial dilution of remedies in which the ratio of the solute to the solvent is 1:99 for each successive stage of dilution. Centesimal potencies of homeopathic remedies are designated either by the numeral alone or by the numeral followed by a small c: 6, 6c, 200, 200c, 10M, 10Mc, etc.

Chronic disease. An illness or symptom of long duration, frequent recurrence, or progressive course of indefinite duration, having no natural tendency to recovery. Opposite of ACUTE DISEASE.

Common symptoms. Symptoms that appear in many cases of disease (e.g., fever) or that appear in diseases of the same character or the same diagnosis.

Constitutional. Relating to the underlying chronic symptoms presented by a patient at any given time, including hereditary factors.

Decimal scale. A system of serial dilution of remedies in which the ratio of the solute to the solvent is 1:9 for each successive stage of dilution; decimal homeopathic potencies are designated by the numeral followed by a small x: 6x, 200x, 10Mx, etc.

Disease entity. A hypothetical construct in orthodox medicine designating a diagnostic category.

Double-blind study. An experimental model in which neither the person conducting the experiment nor the subjects in the experiment know which subjects are being subjected to the condition (or drug) being tested and which are being subjected to a neutral condition (or placebo); an optimum model for studies of the action of drugs.

Drug picture. A compilation of all the information about the effects of a medicine, derived from drug provings, poisonings, and clinical experience.

Dynamization. A process in homeopathy whereby medicines are subjected to serial dilution with succussion to bring out the nonphysical, or dynamic, qualities of the medicine. See POTENTIZATION.

Generals. Symptoms that pertain to the patient as a whole.

Globules. Sugar pills about the size of poppy seeds, used as a vehicle for the administration of homeopathic remedies by moistening them with liquid potencies.

Grading of symptoms. Assigning of relative weights (1 to 3) to the symptoms presented by the patient according to the degree to which the symptoms are marked, the first grade being the most marked and receiving a weight of 3. Similarly, weighting of remedies in the repertory according to the frequency with which they have been noted to produce or cure a given symptom, the most frequent remedies receiving a weight of 3.

Hering's law. A law of cure formulated by Constantine Hering stating that as a patient improves under homeopathic treatment his symptoms will proceed as follows: from within outward, from above downward, from more important to less important organs, and in the reverse order of their appearance.

Holistic. Pertaining to the idea that a whole cannot be analyzed without residue into the sum of its parts.

Homeopathic remedy. A remedy—selected on the basis of the similarity of its symptom picture to the symptom picture of the patient—that demonstrates its similarity by producing a reaction (such as amelioration, aggravation, etc.) in the patient; also, a remedy prepared according to the homeopathic method of potentization.

Iatrogenic. Induced by a physician. Iatrogenic disease is a disease produced by medical treatment.

Indisposition. An illness that is brought on by external stress and that will disappear if the stress is removed.

Isopathy. From the Greek *iso-* ("identical") and *pathein* ("disease, suffering"). Treatment of disease by the use of substances identical to those that produced the disease.

Keynotes. Guideposts, or characteristic symptoms and modalities, pointing to a particular medicine.

Law of similars. The principle that like shall be cured by like, or *Similia similibus curantur.* This principle, recognized by physicians and philosophers since ancient times, became the basis of Hahnemann's formulation of the homeopathic doctrine: the proper remedy for a patient's disease is that substance that is capable of producing, in a healthy person, symptoms similar to those from which the patient suffers.

Materia medica. Latin: "materials of medicine." A collection of detailed descriptions of the symptoms produced and cured by different remedies.

Mentals. Symptoms pertaining to the patient's mind and emotions; classified as GENERALS.

Miasm. An immaterial substance that produces disease by taking hold of the vital force. According to Hahnemann's theory of chronic diseases, a miasm is a way of classifying the patient's signs and symptoms according to a theoretical history of inherited or suppressed chronic disease. The three chronic miasms, according to Hahnemann, are PSORA, SYCOSIS, and SYPHILIS; these three miasms can combine in various ways. Modern homeopaths speak of miasms as distortions of the expression of the vital force, or of the flow of the self-regulating energies of the organism.

Minimum dose. The smallest quantity of a medicine that produces a change in the patient.

Modality. A circumstance that makes the patient or a symptom better or worse; e.g., time of day, temperature, movement, etc.

Nosode. A potentized remedy prepared from such disease material as bacteria, pus, etc.

Organon. Hahnemann's principal work (1810), in which he formulates the doctrine of homeopathy.

Palliation. Alleviation of symptoms without curing the disease that produced them.

Particulars. Symptoms pertaining to individual parts of the body.

Pathogenesis. The production and development of disease; the pathogenesis of a drug is a description of the disease symptoms it produces.

Pathology. Structural and functional changes produced by disease.

Pillule. A sugar tablet used as a vehicle for the administration of homeopathic remedies.

Placebo. From the Latin verb meaning "to please." A medicinally inert substance given for its psychological effect, either to please the patient or as a control in an experiment. In homeopathy, milk sugar, or *saccharum lactis* (lactose) is used as a placebo both in the course of homeopathic treatment and in double-blind provings. The placebo effect is the psychological benefit derived either from the administration of a substance (inert or active) or from the therapeutic set.

Polychrest. From the Greek, meaning "many uses." A remedy whose provings and clinical applications demonstrate that it has many uses.

Potency. A succussed serial dilution of a remedy. *Low potencies* fall within the range of the 3rd, 6th, and 12th serial dilutions; *medium potencies,* the 30th and 200th; and *high potencies,* the 1000th (1M), 50,000th (50M), and upward. The higher the potency, the more dilute is the remedy; the higher potencies are said to be more powerful because they act on a higher dynamic (less physical) plane.

Potentization. The process of serial dilution and succussion by which homeopathic remedies are prepared. Potentization is said to enhance the therapeutic effect of a drug while nullifying its toxic effect.

Primary action. The initial symptom-producing effect of a drug, which—if prescribed according to the Law of Similars—may produce a temporary aggravation of the patient's symptoms.

Proving. A procedure for testing the effects of a substance by administering it to healthy human subjects in order to observe the symptoms it produces.

Psora. A chronic miasm originating with an itching skin eruption (sometimes equated with scabies) which, by being suppressed through allopathic drugging, is driven inward and expresses itself in varied functional and physical symptoms. According to Hahnemann, psora is transmissible through heredity as well as through infection and is the basis of seven-eighths of man's diseases.

Remedy. In homeopathy, a medicine administered according to the Law of Similars.

Remedy epidemicus. A remedy that has been determined, on the basis of the Law of Similars, to be curative in an epidemic disease.

Repertorization. The process of matching a patient's symptoms to the remedies that can produce and cure them; this is done by means of a REPERTORY in order to arrive at the single remedy that most closely matches the patient's total symptom picture.

Repertory. An index to symptoms that lists the remedies that have produced each symptom or have been shown to cure it.

Rubric. A symptom used as a heading in a repertory; the rubric is followed by a list of medicines that can produce this symptom in a healthy person or relieve this symptom in the sick.

Saccharum lactis. Abbreviation: *Sac. lac.* Lactose, or milk sugar; used as a diluent in preparing triturations of medicines, as a vehicle for the administration of liquid potencies, and as a placebo.

Secondary action. A second set of symptoms that appear following the administration of a drug, produced by the reaction of the organism against the drug's initial effect. If the drug has been prescribed according to the Law of Similars, the secondary action consists of a stimulation of the reactive vital force and an amelioration of the patient's presenting symptoms.

Side effects. Effects of a drug other than the effect it was administered to evoke.

Simillimum. Latin: "most similar." The medicine that most closely matches the totality of the patient's symptoms (on the basis of the Law of Similars) and that will give the greatest relief.

Strange, rare, and peculiar symptom. An unusual symptom, peculiar to a particular medicine.

Succussion. Forceful shaking, as in the preparation of liquid potencies of homeopathic remedies.

Susceptibility. Sensitivity to a disease; also, sensitivity to a particular remedy owing to a disturbance of the vital force as reflected in the total symptom picture, which resembles the symptom picture of the remedy.

Sycosis. The chronic miasmatic form of gonorrhea, whose chronic symptoms are characterized by overgrowth of tissue (hair, skin, etc.).

Symptoms. Observable changes in the mental, emotional, and physical condition of a patient, resulting from a derangement of the vital force.

Syphilis. The chronic miasm arising from suppressed or inherited syphilis, whose symptoms are characterized by destruction of tissue.

Tincture. An alcoholic solution of a medicinal substance.

Trituration. Reduction of a solid substance to a fine powder by grinding with mortar and pestle.

Vis medicatrix naturae. Latin: the "healing force of nature."

Vital force. The intangible energy that animates all living creatures and mediates their physical, emotional, and mental responses to external stress. When the vital force is in balance, there is health; when it is out of balance, there is disease.

INDEX

ABOUT THE AUTHORS

Michael A. Weiner earned his Bachelor of Science degree at the City University of New York, M.S. and M.A. degrees in medical botany and medical anthropology from the University of Hawaii; and a doctorate in Nutritional Enthnomedicine from the University of California at Berkeley. He has received numerous honors and grants, including three from the National Science Foundation and one from the National Cancer Institute. His writings have appeared in many scientifi journals, most recently in *The New England Journal of Medicine.* He is the author of fourteen books including such best sellers as *Earth Medicine-Earth Foods* and *Maximum Immunity.* Dr. Weiner is presently Director of Research for the National Arthritis Institute.

Kathleen Goss is a writer, researcher and editor who is committed to the ongoing revolution in health and consciousness, and who uses her scholarly skills to interpret nonorthodox points of view for a popular audience. With Dr. Weiner she has also co-authored *The Art of Feeding Children Well.* She lives in San Francisco.